Choice, information and dignity

Involving users and carers in care
management in mental health

John Carpenter and Silvia Sbaraini

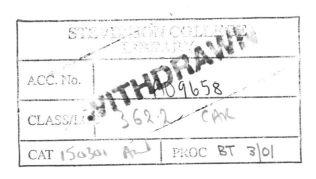
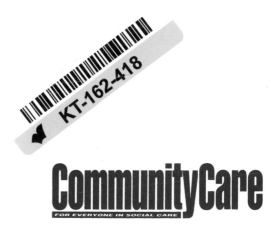
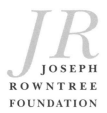

JOSEPH
ROWNTREE
FOUNDATION

CommunityCare
FOR EVERYONE IN SOCIAL CARE

First published in Great Britain in 1997 by
The Policy Press
University of Bristol
Rodney Lodge
Grange Road
Bristol BS8 4EA
Telephone: (0117) 973 8797
Fax: (0117) 973 7308
E-mail: tpp@bris.ac.uk
Website: http://www.bris.ac.uk/Publications/TPP

ISBN 1 86134 069 9

The *Community Care into Practice* series has been established by *Community Care* and the Joseph Rowntree Foundation to make research available in the social care field to a wide audience of managers and practitioners.

Community Care is the leading magazine in the field of social care. It has supported this report as part of its commitment to debate and the dissemination of information.

The report was written by John Carpenter, Centre for Applied Social Studies, University of Durham and Silvia Sbaraini, The Tizard Centre, University of Kent.

The Joseph Rowntree Foundation has supported this project as part of its programme of research and innovative development projects, which it hopes will be of value to policy makers and practitioners. The facts presented and views expressed in this report, however, are those of the authors and not necessarily those of the Foundation.

The Policy Press is working to counter discrimination on grounds of gender, race, disability, age and sexuality.

Designed by Adkins Design
Printed by Hobbs the Printers Ltd, Southampton

Contents

Acknowledgements

We would particularly like to thank all the users and carers involved in this project who helped to design the approach and the evaluation, acted as interviewers, answered questions or responded to questionnaires.

Jill Butler, voluntary services officer, and Pam Wood, secretary for the Voluntary Services Bureau organised the coding and posting of the questionnaires. The evaluation would not have been possible without their generous help.

Jean Evans, social worker in Thanet, assisted (as part of her work for a MSc degree at the Institute of Psychiatry) with the development of Goal Attainment Scales and Quality of Life questionnaires for some of the users.

We would also like to thank the staff of Canterbury and Thanet Community Healthcare Trust and of Canterbury and Thanet Area of Kent Social Services Department, managers and practitioners, who cooperated in the implementation of the approach. We hope that the encouraging results reported here will encourage them further in their efforts to involve and empower users and carers in mental healthcare.

Finally, we wish to express our thanks to the members of the project advisory group for their consistently wise and constructive advice and, not least, for their encouragement, especially when the obstacles seemed overwhelming.

Project advisory group
Lisa Barcan, service user, London
Claire Benjamin, project adviser, Joseph Rowntree Trust
Dr Ian Bennun, district psychologist, South Devon Community Healthcare Trust; senior lecturer in clinical psychology, University of Exeter
Maggie Gallant, development worker, FURST project Thanet; service user
Elaine Haughie, research and development officer, Kent County Council Social Services
Azad Mohammedaly, quality/business manager, Canterbury and Thanet Community Healthcare Trust

Justine Schneider, research fellow, Personal Social Services Research Unit, University of Kent at Canterbury; non-executive member, East Kent Health Authority
Paul Taylor, locality manager, mental health, Kent County Council Social Services Department
Pat Thompson, chair, Canterbury and Faversham Branch of National Schizophrenia Fellowship; carer
Barbara Webb, project liaison officer, Joseph Rowntree Trust
Dr Steven Wood, consultant psychiatrist and medical director, Canterbury and Thanet Community Healthcare Trust; honorary senior lecturer, United Medical and Dental Schools, University of London

Research team
John Carpenter, senior lecturer in applied psychology of mental health, Tizard Centre, University of Kent (now professor of applied social studies, University of Durham)
Silvia Sbaraini, research associate, Tizard Centre, University of Kent
Enid Skene, Pat Thompson, Paul Salako, Rachel Epps, Brian Campbell, research interviewers
Barbara Duce, research secretary, Tizard Centre, University of Kent

Summary

Can mental health services be more responsive to the needs of people with severe and long-term mental health problems? Is it possible to involve service users and their carers effectively in developing plans for their care and treatment in the community? This report describes the development of an integrated approach to care management and care programming, which aimed specifically to involve users and carers. The evaluation found that:

- Having a care programme had a positive influence on users' views and experiences of services. Users with care programmes felt more involved in planning their own care and treatment, had more choice and were better informed about rights and services.

- Users with a care programme were more likely to have been asked whether they wanted a carer involved in planning their care and to report that their carer had discussed their care with mental health professionals.

- Over three quarters of users agreed with their care programmes, thought that they were clear and comprehensive and that they addressed their needs. Two thirds considered that their care programme had worked out well, or very well.

- The positive effect of a care programme on users' views and experiences was consistent across time; users with a care programme continued to feel more involved and to have more choice in their care treatment.

- There were some indications that a shortage of resources in terms of staff time and facilities, especially for work, inhibited choice for some users.

- Both users and carers were positive about their relationships with care managers - building up a stable, trusting relationship with one professional enhanced service delivery and continuity.

- Initially, three quarters of users wanted their carers involved in planning their care, but six months later, users were less likely to report that their carers were involved; they were also less likely to want them involved.

- Carers wanted to be involved in their relatives' care. Carers whose relatives had care programmes tended to be more positive in their views of services. However, carers tended to feel less involved after the initial care programme meetings.

- Carers' own needs were rarely addressed by services.

- Most mental health professionals were committed to the philosophy of the Care Programme Approach and were very positive about its effects on assessing and monitoring users' needs. They considered that it had a positive effect on users' involvement with their own care and most thought that it had a positive impact on involving carers. Over half thought it benefited multidisciplinary team working.

- Over half the professionals thought the process very time consuming and over 80% thought that it was difficult, or very difficult, to implement within existing resources.

- Only half the GPs in the area who responded to a survey believed they knew what a care programme was, and 90% had not attended either a care programme planning or review meeting. However, over 60% said they would be willing to attend such meetings if they had time and/or were paid.

- Over half the GPs supported the principle of involving users in developing care programmes, and nearly three quarters agreed with the involvement of family carers.

1
Introduction and overview

Can mental health services be more responsive to the needs of people with severe and or long-term mental health problems? Is it possible to involve service users and their carers in developing plans for their care and treatment in the community? Can users be empowered by this process? Will it enable them to achieve their goals and lead to improvements in the quality of their lives?

This report describes the development and evaluation of a project specifically designed to involve and empower users of mental health services and their carers. It concerns involvement at an *individual* level in the process of 'care management': assessing needs, developing, and implementing a plan of care, monitoring and review.

The project took place in an ordinary mental health service in South East England in an area with levels of psychiatric morbidity close to the national average. During the running of the project no special funding was available; on the contrary, the service was under particular pressure from a shortage of psychiatric hospital places and specialist staff. The lessons from the project should therefore be widely applicable to other mental health services.

The project is an example of *participatory research*. The approach, and its evaluation, were designed in collaboration with service users and carers and they also acted as research interviewers and as members of the project advisory group. Other 'stakeholders', mental health professionals and managers from health and social services, took part in the design and interpretation of the results. As they became available, the results were fed back to the services and to user groups throughout the project. This prompted management action to improve the implementation of the approach and to secure additional resources to make it more effective.

The project is a rare example of an attempt to *evaluate* user involvement empirically. The methods used were both quantitative (surveys, questionnaires and scales which could be analysed statistically and used to compare groups) and qualitative (interviews, questionnaires and case studies, which add a richness to the data collected).

The report begins with an introduction to user involvement and care management and the Care Programme Approach (CPA) in mental health. The development of the CPA in the project area is then described and this is followed by a discussion of issues in its implementation. The results of two surveys of mental health professionals' views and a survey of the opinions of general practitioners are presented.

The methods used to evaluate users' and carers' experiences, including the use of 'peer interviewing', are described and the results presented. A comparison is made between those users who had received a care programme and those who had not, and a number of significant differences are revealed. For example, users with a care programme were more likely to feel that they had been able to take an active part in working out a plan with professionals for their care and treatment and that they had more choice. This provides evidence of the effectiveness of the Approach. The opinions of family carers are also reported. These indicate that carers also felt positive about the Approach and were involved in their relatives' care. Users and carers were followed up six months later. Once again, the results showed the benefits of having a care programme in that users felt more involved and had more choice. Most users felt that their care programmes had worked out well, although for some the results were mixed and a small minority had become disillusioned. This range of outcomes is illustrated in a series of case profiles of service users and their carers.

The main findings are summarised throughout the report in a series of boxes and the report concludes with a discussion and policy implications.

2
User involvement in mental health services

Hearing the voices of the users of mental health services

In 1992, Peter Campbell, who describes himself as a 'survivor' of mental health services, commented on the effects of moves towards consumerism in government policies concerning health and social care. He wrote:

> Whereas five years ago it felt revolutionary for a survivor to stand up at a public meeting and ask for choice, information and dignity within services, such demands are now considered reasonable requests. Addressing such desires still seems to require enormous and apparently painful contortions within the service system and those who direct it. But voicing such desires no longer seems to be seen as a symptom of malicious intent. (Campbell, 1992, p 118)

This report describes and evaluates a project which was designed to promote choice, provide information and enhance the dignity of people with severe and/or long-term mental health problems who are receiving treatment and care from the statutory services. It includes a description of the 'contortions' within the service during the implementation of the project and identifies a number of lessons for developments in mainstream services elsewhere.

The evaluation was supported by a grant from the Joseph Rowntree Foundation, whose community care division had invited proposals for the evaluation of user involvement. There is plenty of research which identifies the limitations of current practice (eg, Ellis, 1993; Lindow and Morris, 1995) and many examples of schemes designed to promote user involvement (eg, Marsh and Fisher, 1992), but little in the way of *evaluation* of such schemes. (A notable exception is Holly and Webb, 1993.) We hope that this report will make a contribution to the literature, in terms of both its findings and the methods used.

An important part of the project was to involve service users and carers in both the development and the evaluation. Thus, users and carers were part of the group which identified the project goals and objectives and designed the Approach. They also helped to develop the evaluation questionnaires and conducted interviews with fellow users and carers. Users and carers were also members of the project advisory group and contributed their ideas to discussions about the management of the evaluation and the interpretation of its results.

User involvement in community care

In its guidance on the community care changes at the beginning of the 1990s, the Department of Health (DoH) promoted the concept of user involvement in the planning, delivery and evaluation of services at both an individual and a service level. At an individual level this was seen as being achieved through the process of care management. The objectives of care management as described in the guidance include:

- treating users with respect
- promoting individual choice and self-determination, and
- promoting partnership between users, carers and service providers. (DoH, 1990, p 23)

Care management in mental health

The care (or 'case') management approach was first developed in mental health services in the United States (Onyett, 1992). Various models have been described and evaluated, all of which were founded on the conviction that the coordination of a range of services, delivered to an individual by a number of different agencies and professionals, can be more effectively achieved where responsibility lies with an identified care manager.

In Britain, encouraging results of three case management demonstration projects have been published (Muijen et al, 1992; Merson et al, 1992; Burns et al, 1993). However, this research has been done in 'centres of excellence' and there remains a need for information which can assist care managers working under the ordinary conditions prevailing in mental health services in Britain, including very much larger caseloads. This point is particularly important because the government has already required the health service to implement a form of care management, the Care Programme Approach (CPA), without providing any extra resources.

The Care Programme Approach and user involvement

The CPA came into being because the government was concerned about inadequate follow-up care for people leaving psychiatric hospitals, as evident in a number of widely publicised scandals. The DoH made a requirement that health trusts, in collaboration with social services departments, design and implement jointly agreed systems for care management of the users of specialist mental health services (DoH, 1990). It is important to note that while the government did not prescribe how the CPA would work, the circular nevertheless emphasised various elements of good practice, including:

- systematic assessment of the user's health and social care needs by a multidisciplinary team
- an agreed plan of care and treatment
- the allocation of a 'key worker' with responsibility for maintaining contact and monitoring the implementation of the plan
- regular reviews of the user's progress.

The importance of involving patients (sic) and carers was particularly stressed in the original guidance:

> It is important that proper opportunities are provided for patients themselves to take part in discussions about their proposed care programmes, so that they have the chance to discuss different treatment possibilities and agree the programme to be implemented. (DoH, 1990)

Similarly, the DoH recognised that relatives and other carers often know a great deal about the user's life, interests and abilities as well as having personal experience of the user's illness (sic) over many years. Consequently,

> Wherever consistent with the patient's wishes, professional staff should seek to involve them [the carers] in the planning and subsequent oversight of community care and treatment. (DoH, 1990)

Further, if a care programme depends on support from a carer,

... it should be agreed in advance with the carer, who should be properly advised about such aspects of the patient's care as necessary.

In addition, professional staff may be able to offer the carer help in coming to terms with his/her role vis-à-vis the patient. (DoH, 1990)

Further guidance on the CPA was given in successive editions of the *Key area handbook on mental health* issued in support of the Health of the Nation initiative (DoH, 1993; 1994). Most recently, in November 1995, the DoH issued *Building bridges, a guide to arrangements for inter-agency working for the care and protection of severely mentally ill people.* This document emphasised that the "CPA is the cornerstone of the Government's mental health policy" (DoH, 1995, sec 3.0.3). Further, it reiterated, in bold type, the importance of involving service users and carers in care programming: **"Users and carers must be involved"** (DoH, 1995, sec 1.3.6).

As we shall see, putting this intention into practice is not a straightforward matter. Early research into the operation of the CPA commissioned by the DoH noted only minimal involvement of users and carers (North, Ritchie and Ward, 1993; Schneider et al, 1993). For example, they rarely received copies of assessments or attended reviews. The only practice geared towards participation observed with any frequency was the requirement that the service user sign the care programme. However, as the researchers observed, such requirements can be ineffectual if they are not reinforced with genuine consultation. A survey by the Social Services Inspectorate concluded that,

> With one or two notable exceptions, the involvement of users and carers was very limited. Many users and carers felt disadvantaged. They were not aware of their entitlements.... Nor were they aware of the resources and service options that might have enabled them to make better choices.... (Social Services Inspectorate/DoH, 1995)

The finding that, in spite of government exhortations, users had only token involvement in planning their own care is hardly surprising. Mental health user groups have long protested against their disempowerment by the psychiatric system (Berforth et al, 1990). The MIND/Roehampton Institute 'People First' survey of over 500 users who had had at least one hospital admission found that only 20% were satisfied with the information they were given by psychiatrists about their treatment (Rogers and Pilgrim, 1991). Similarly, a study by Hansson found that even where there was generally high satisfaction with regard to staff-user relationships, treatment programmes and the physical environment, users were dissatisfied with the information they were given and their lack of influence on their management and the design of treatment (Hansson, 1989). Eighty-two per cent were dissatisfied with the lack of information about the possibility of reading their case records, over 40% with information about their mental health problems, and over 50% with the amount of consideration given to their own views about treatment.

The Care Programme Approach and social services care management

The government intended the CPA to apply to 'all people in contact with specialist mental health services'. In practice, at the start of the project, the national picture according to the Audit Commission was that it was being used for a restricted group of people with more severe problems (Audit Commission, 1994). These included people compulsorily or repeatedly admitted to hospital, those needing continuing residential care and those considered to be 'at risk' in the community. These service users almost inevitably have complex social care needs and therefore come within the scope of the social services departments' responsibilities under the community care legislation to provide assessment and care management (DoH, 1993). The two approaches are therefore complementary and, as recommended in *Building bridges,* in some parts of the country, including the study area, an integrated approach has been developed (DoH, 1995).

3
Developing an approach

This chapter describes how professionals and managers worked together with users and carers to develop and implement the CPA. The project took place in a health trust and social services district in South East England. The area includes two main population centres, a cathedral city which is a major tourist centre and university town, and seaside towns which double in population during the summer months. The latter area is designated as an area of special assisted status by the European Union (EU) (one of only four in the country) because unemployment rates are so high. (The area has a population of 300,000. The Mental Illness Needs Index [MINI] scores of social deprivation factors known to be linked to mental illness varies between 98.5 for the cathedral city and 104.6 for the seaside towns.) There is a large number of former psychiatric patients from the London area living in the seaside towns.

The Victorian asylum serving the area was finally closed in 1994. There are now two inpatient units and four community mental health teams with long stay residential care being provided by the voluntary and independent sectors. (The total annual budget for the trust is £41.3m, of which £7.5m is spent on adult mental health services: £4.8m on inpatient services; £2.7m on community-based schemes.)

The project began in 1993 when one of us was working for one half day a week with members of a community mental health team in order to help them develop skills in work with users with severe and/or long-term mental health problems and their families. A rudimentary form of care programming had been introduced within the health service two years earlier and a very much more complex assessment system using an elaborate proforma had been given to social services staff following the implementation of the Community Care Act. However, there was little evidence that these two systems were being used. A sample of care programmes provided by team members was examined. What was most apparent here was great variation in approach, including the use of different forms (most of which were partially completed check lists of 'services to be delivered').

Working with the multidisciplinary team

An assessment of current practice in involving users and carers was carried out by attending ward rounds in the hospital and meetings in the community between users and staff, including psychiatrists, psychiatric nurses, social workers and occupational therapists. Although staff were sympathetic to the *idea* of involving users and carers in planning the user's own care and empowering them to take greater control over their own lives, they often lacked the knowledge and sometimes the skills to make this a reality. Further, users had very little idea of what choices might be available and tended passively to accept the professional's recommendation for the 'appropriate' treatment or service (eg, "You need to develop your social skills - go to the day hospital."). Subsequent interviews with service users revealed that they felt unable to exercise choice or even to complain if they did not agree with the care programme offered. Family carers complained that they were given little or no information about diagnosis or treatment but were expected to pick up the pieces when their relative was sent home.

These views were reported to the mental health team members and their respective managers in health and social services who agreed to take part in a development project designed to make the aspiration of user and carer involvement a reality. Fortunately, the respective managers had already agreed in principle to use a joint approach for both statutory tasks, CPA and care management, including an agreement to use the same eligibility criteria.

Two half-day workshops were held with the 15 members of the team, during which the principles and practice of involving users and carers in assessing and planning mental healthcare were discussed and the team members' commitment to the project sought. Most team members, with the exception of the consultant psychiatrist, took part. It was clear that staff were in sympathy with the goal of increasing user and carer involvement in planning the user's own care and empowering them to take greater control over their own lives. Indeed, these goals were explicitly stated in the team's 'mission statement' as a preamble to the operational policy, which they had jointly agreed. Most team members were willing to accept that there was scope for improvement in their existing practice and to discuss their own ideas about achieving user and carer involvement so that these might be fed into the development of a better system.

Involving stakeholders

Representatives of those identified as having a stake in the service (the 'stakeholders') were invited to a further workshop at the University. Participants were:

- service users (members of the local user forum)
- carers (members of the local branch of the National Schizophrenia Fellowship)
- nursing and social worker community mental health team members
- senior managers in health and social services
- a GP, and
- staff of the inpatient psychiatric unit.

The initial task was defined as being to identify attributes of good practice in involving users and carers. The question posed was: "What would have to happen if users and carers were to be fully involved in planning the user's mental healthcare?"

Box 1: What service users wanted

Service users wanted professionals to:

- listen to and appreciate users' views on what they felt about being referred to the mental health services and/or admitted to hospital

- listen to and understand their problems and needs - not simply make a diagnosis

- discuss ideas about treatment and care

- provide information about services and rights, so that they could make informed choices

- provide information about medication and its side effects and discuss alternatives, try to involve family and carers - if the user wanted this.

> # Box 2: What carers wanted
> Carers wanted professionals to:
>
> - listen to their opinions on the user's problems and needs - they usually knew most about the user
>
> - provide information about the user's psychiatric status and medication
>
> - offer advice on how to manage difficult behaviour
>
> - provide information about rights and services, including access to emergency services and respite care
>
> - discuss what support the carer might be willing to give, and not take such support for granted
>
> - consider the carer's own needs.

There was discussion about possible conflicts between users and family carers and whether next of kin were entitled to information. It was clarified that if users specifically ask that their family or carers not be involved, then their wishes must be respected - unless the family/carers have been appointed by a court to manage the user's affairs or if there is a 'public interest' ground for giving them information (eg, if the user is threatening violence). In addition, under the 1983 Mental Health Act, approved social workers have a duty to inform the nearest relative if a user is being considered for compulsory detention in hospital, or has already been detained.

The working group of users, carers, professionals and managers agreed that the first outcome of a participatory approach should be a written care programme, an open document circulated to all involved parties, as agreed by the user. (A written care programme is required by government guidance [DoH, 1995, sec 3.1]. This document also advises that copies of the care programme be sent to all those present at the care planning meeting and any other relevant parties, "subject to the need to maintain an appropriate level of confidentiality" [sec 3.1.14].)

Further, a care plan which had been *devised in collaboration with user and carers should contain,* among other information, the following elements:

Box 3: Ingredients of a care programme
The care programme should contain:

- user's views on: referral and/or admission to hospital; problems, needs; goals; involvement of carers and family

- carers' views: support they are able to provide to user; if relevant, carers' own needs and arrangements for planning to meet them

- information given to users and carers on rights and services, including medication

- evidence of choices given; purpose of interventions described in terms of problems/needs/goals (is it clear how the intervention will meet the need?)

- explicit agreements; monitoring and review arrangements and recording of any unmet need.

By this time, it had become apparent that the existing care programme and care management procedures and forms would have to be completely revised if the CPA was to achieve the above objectives. The service managers agreed with this proposal and that one of the four mental health teams would pilot a new approach to the CPA which took user and carer involvement seriously. We term this the Approach.

Form and procedures
Through consultation with the group of stakeholders, a set of procedures and written records was developed. The key features were:

Box 4: Features of the Approach

- convening care planning and review meetings involving users, carers (family, friends, or care staff from residential homes), an independent advocate (if requested) and professionals

- recording users' and carers' views on their involvement with mental health services and admission to hospital

- identifying and recording separately the user's, carers' and professionals' views on problems and needs, and aims, and noting disagreements

- formulating action plans designed to meet needs (rather than to use those services which happened to exist locally) and agreeing a 'contract', including monitoring and review arrangements

- providing specific information about rights and services, including medication and how to complain

- explicit agreement (by signature) of all parties.

A leaflet was prepared giving specific guidelines for community mental health team members, whether from health or social services, on arranging care programme meetings and developing care programmes. Further guidance was developed on conducting reviews.

'Your care programme', an information leaflet in question and answer form, was designed for service users. The leaflet explained the purpose of the care programme and emphasised the importance and value of users' participation. A parallel leaflet, 'Care programmes. A guide for carers' was also produced.

A CPA form (see Appendix B) was designed in the light of the objectives shown in Box 3. It consisted of a number of sections:

1. Basic information about the service user (client) and carer (family or professional carer), names and addresses of care manager, psychiatrist, GP and other involved individuals and agencies.

2. Information on the user's and carers' views on their involvement with mental health services.

3. A check list of needs/problems to be considered in the assessment.

4. Information about medication, including prescribing and injection arrangements.

5. Arrangements for monitoring and review of the care programme.

6. A check list of information on rights and services.

7. An opportunity for user, carer and care manager to sign their agreement to the care programme.

In addition, for each problem or need identified in the assessment, there was a separate sheet for recording detailed information about the user's, carers' and professionals' respective views on the nature of the problem or need, their aims, action to be taken, and by whom. Finally, there was space to record 'unmet' need(s). (See example, Appendix B.) A review form and continuation sheets were designed using a similar format.

Box 5: User guide to care programme

Your care programme

Before you leave hospital, we want to talk with you about any help that you may need once you have left. We would like to work with you to draw up a plan to meet any continuing health and social care needs you may have. We call this a 'care programme'. This leaflet explains what it means and tries to answer some questions. If you have any other questions, please ask.

What is it about?

First of all, we want to listen to what you have to say. We want to be sure that we know what you think about the following:

*   being admitted to hospital and plans for your discharge
*   your problems and needs and what your goals are
*   what to do about your problems
*   what help you would like to have from family, carers and professionals.

Then we want to:

*   agree with you a plan of action - who is going to do what and when.

Note: Although we think that having a care programme is the best way to organise your care, it is not compulsory. If you are not happy with the idea, tell your key worker or key nurse.

Who will be involved?

You, of course, and, with your agreement, your family or carers. Your 'key nurse' - the nurse on the ward who has been taking a special interest in you. A 'key worker', a community nurse, occupational therapist, social worker or social services care manager who will be responsible for organising your care once you leave hospital. Your doctor or other professionals involved in your care may wish to come to the meeting if there is something special they way to say, especially if you are on 'section' or if there are questions about your medication.

If you have been living in a residential or nursing home, it might be a good idea for someone from the home to come along to see that they know how best to help you. But this is up to you. You may invite anyone else who you think could help and support you.

How will it happen?

Your key worker or key nurse will discuss with you who should come and then arrange a meeting as soon as is convenient. It will normally take place on the ward and will usually last between 45 minutes to one hour. Your care manager will make sure your views are recorded on a form and everyone will discuss a plan of care for you.

You will get a copy of the form later. Once you have read it, you will be asked to sign it to show that you agree. If the key nurse or your key worker has misunderstood something, you can ask them to change it. With your agreement, the form will be sent to your GP and to others involved in your care so that everyone knows what is going on. You will have your own copy to keep.

What happens when you leave hospital?

Your key worker will be responsible for seeing that your care programme is carried out. They will meet you and, with your agreement, your carers, to check that everything is going OK. At agreed intervals they will review your programme with you and make sure that it is still meeting your needs. If any new problems have arisen, a new care programme will be worked out.

What if you are not happy with your care programme?

Then please tell your key nurse or key worker straight away. We want to give you the best possible service, so you have to tell us if we are not getting it right. If your key nurse or key worker does not seem interested or you do not think they are taking you seriously, then you have a right to complain.

4
Ideas into practice

Within the pilot area, a monthly professional development group was established. An audit approach was to be used, the aim of which was agreed as being, 'to improve practice in involving service users and carers in care programming.' Team members discussed the set of quality indicators and agreed that these should form the basis for an audit of completed care programmes. The forms were analysed according to the indicators and the results presented for discussion every three months.

Monthly one-hour discussion groups were held to identify strengths and weaknesses and to review particular case examples. The objective was to devise ways of overcoming difficulties and improving practice. In addition, the facilitator took part in some 12 care programmes and review meetings in users' homes, health centres and hospital wards.

User participation
These professional development group meetings identified issues concerning participation in, and arrangements for care programming meetings. One concern was with users in hospital who were too ill and/or unhappy to want to take part in meetings. This posed a particular problem when the user was detained compulsorily under the terms of Mental Health Act which requires multidisciplinary 'Section 117' meetings to be held within a few days of admission. In these cases, it was agreed that a short, formal meeting be held in order to meet the statutory requirements and to identify the professionals' concerns and to allocate responsibilities. This would be followed later by the CPA meeting. It was accepted that meetings worked best when the care manager (community psychiatric nurse or social worker) and the key worker (the patient's 'named nurse' on the ward) understood the principles behind the approach and how they had been incorporated in the design of the form. Care managers also needed to be well briefed on services and rights (eg, Citizen Advocacy and access to records).

Not surprisingly, users sometimes needed reassurance and encouragement that they really could express their views. However, once they got the idea that the professionals were genuinely interested, most played an active part. The procedure whereby users are asked to state their needs *first* seemed particularly valuable in helping them take some control of the proceedings. Of course, both carer and care manager had a chance to disagree or add new concerns because the form allowed everyone's different views to be discussed and recorded. This seemed useful even for users detained in hospital under Section of the Mental Health Act even if they had no power, they could at least request an explanation from the consultant psychiatrist.

It was apparent that professionals did not always find it easy to move from a *diagnosis-led* approach ("He's got schizophrenia. He needs medication.") or a *service-led* approach ("She looks like a suitable candidate for Jane's group. I'll refer her."). A *needs-led* approach required the identification of the need or problem first and then discussion of possible solutions. Further, the users and carers had to understand the relationship between their particular problem or need and the proposed intervention.

From a review of the CPA forms, it was also apparent that some professionals found it difficult to grasp the importance of recording the *user's* own views of their problems/needs - even though the form explicitly asked for these. What was recorded in many instances was obviously the *professional's* view (eg, "Sheila [name used for example only] needs to take medication", rather than, for example, "I want the voices to go away").

Advantages and disadvantages

The development group meetings also provided an opportunity to identify the advantages and disadvantages of the approach from the perspective of the care managers.

> ## Box 6: Advantages of involving users and carers: care managers' views
>
> - stimulating comments and feedback from users
> - providing a clear focus for assessment and planning
> - highlighting reasons for referral to other agencies
> - providing users and carers with information about rights and services
> - explaining reasons for medication and possible side-effects
> - identifying clearly the different views of users, carers, and key workers on problems and needs
> - revealing lots of useful and relevant information
> - identifying clearly that users can take responsibility and do things for themselves
> - encouraging the contributions of family members.

The main *disadvantage* perceived by staff was that the process took more time than previously. The assessment and planning meetings themselves took up between 45 minutes and one-and-a-half hours, depending on the amount of preparatory work which had been done, the complexity of the user's needs and their ability to contribute to the discussion. In some cases this was longer than the participants and care manager had allowed. To this must be added the time involved explaining the purpose and procedures to the user, liaising with carers and other professionals, and in setting up the meetings themselves. Following the meetings, the forms had to be written out clearly for typing, typed, checked with the user and distributed. In the event that the user's condition had deteriorated severely, or for some other reason the care programme had proved difficult to implement, all the preceding work could sometimes be seen by the care manager as time wasted.

Some care managers expressed concern that if users understood their rights, they might decline to accept medical treatment that psychiatrists and other mental health professionals considered they needed; this, they feared could result in the user's mental health deteriorating and their being readmitted to hospital. Indeed this was said to have been the outcome in at least one case. A related worry on the part of some professionals was for users who "lacked insight into their illness", had unrealistic aspirations or were "unable to cope". These staff questioned the assumption that people with mental illness could act rationally and that it was actually oppressive practice to treat them as if they could. This was, however, a minority view, though strongly held.

Training in the Approach

During 1995, this approach to care programming was implemented in the three other community mental health teams for adults and two for older people. A training programme was devised with the following learning objectives:

Box 7: Learning objectives for a joint training programme

1. Understand the background to the CPA and its three key elements: multidisciplinary input; community key worker maintaining contact; involving users and carers.

2. Appreciate the reasons for involving users and carers.

3. Understand the relationship between CPA, care management, Section 117 procedures and the Supervision Register.

4. Recognise the limitations of current practice (and dispel complacency - "We're doing it all already.").

5. Understand procedures, forms, and leaflets.

6. Develop an appreciation of, and skills in, needs-led assessment and care planning.

7. Cultivate skills in encouraging the participation of users and carers, involving them in the process, and enabling their empowerment.

Learning together

The framework for the training programme consisted of an initial presentation of the project to each team in order to elicit their agreement. In accordance with the philosophy of the approach, the professionals were asked to agree to service users and carers taking part in the training sessions and invitations were extended to the user forum and to a carers group. Understandably, there was some suspicion among some members on each side, but in the event four carers and ten users attended the workshops in two team areas.

The half-day workshops aimed to cover objectives 1 to 5 in Box 7. Each workshop began with a presentation about the CPA and a discussion about the advantages of involving users and carers. The contributions of users and carers to this discussion were very constructive. The CPA procedures and forms were explained and participants, working in small mixed groups, were invited to discuss a fictional case example. They were asked to assess the needs of a user from the perspectives of the user, carer and professionals and to agree on a course of action. The case example (Appendix C) was written to illustrate contradictory views on problems and needs and to simulate some of the difficulties which might be encountered in involving users and carers.

Community and inpatient staff were then encouraged to work together in pairs in order to make a joint assessment and develop a care programme for an eligible service user, involving the carer, if appropriate. It was hoped that by the time of the second workshop, approximately two months later, most members of the team would have had the experience of developing a care programme. The focus of this workshop could then be on resolving any problems and clarifying procedures, and on skills development (objectives 6 and 7) through reflecting on practice and problem-based learning. This, it was hoped, would set a pattern for peer group supervision linked to clinical audit. A third workshop introduced the system for reviews and outlined the procedures to be employed by the researchers in the evaluation of the project.

If users are to be involved as participants in the CPA, they could benefit from training as well. Consequently, we also gave a presentation to well attended meetings of the local users' forum at which we explained the principles of the CPA and discussed the procedures which were being adopted.

5
Implementing the Approach

We aimed to monitor the implementation of the Approach in the four areas through attending meetings of health and social services managers and team leaders and by auditing the care programmes which had been developed. We asked professionals in two of the areas to complete a questionnaire concerning their views on the CPA during one of the initial training sessions. We followed them up six months later, inviting them to give their views in the light of their experience of its implementation. We also conducted a survey of all GPs in the areas to seek their opinions on the CPA and attitudes to user involvement. Finally, we surveyed and interviewed users and carers in order to assess the outcomes of the Approach from their perspectives; this is the subject of the following two chapters.

Managers' meetings
The managers' meetings were generally effective in identifying problems with procedures and practice and developing solutions. There were initial difficulties in the relationships between ward and community staff (which required that the roles of the key worker and care manager be redefined) and problems in involving consultant psychiatrists in meetings. The meetings have continued to monitor developments. (During 1994/95, there was a significant change in government requirements about the CPA. It had originally been intended to apply to *all* people in contact with specialist mental health services but this had been widely judged by health trusts as unworkable. The DoH responded by recommending the 'tiered CPA', a system of levels of intervention and professional involvement depending on the 'complexity' of the user's needs [DoH, 1995, sec 2.3]. A tiered system was subsequently devised for the area and formally adopted in August 1996. This system retains some features of the original approach, including space for recording users' and carers' views about involvement, but others, notably the opportunity to record separate views about problems, needs and goals, have been omitted in the interests of producing a more streamlined document. The focus of this evaluation has remained on users with 'complex needs'.)

There was a commitment to interagency working on the part of both health and social services colleagues, although this was clearly put under strain by distortions in the pattern of service provision as a result of the influence of GP fundholders on the health trust and of the social services department's changing eligibility criteria. Thus GP fundholders sought contracts with the trust which increasingly drew the community psychiatric nurses into counselling work within their own surgeries and away from work in the mental health teams. On the other hand, the social workers were required by their department to focus almost entirely on people with enduring mental health problems. Furthermore, during this time the service as whole was under enormous pressure: a report by the District Audit, an arm of the Audit Commission, identified the area as having one of the highest psychiatric bed occupancy rates in the country (170%), community psychiatric nurses with considerably higher than average caseloads and less than half the recommended number of consultant psychiatrists (District Audit, 1995). The same report, incidentally, had described the CPA system as "excellent" and had observed that it, "places the service user firmly at the centre of the service." On the other hand, it noted deficiencies in multidisciplinary assessment which the managers have sought to rectify through making firm arrangements for care programme meetings in order to ensure the participation of psychiatrists.

Audit reports

We had agreed with the managers to provide regular reports based on an analysis of the care programme forms, giving descriptive information about the number of care programmes completed, the characteristics of the users concerned, the identity of the care managers, other professionals involved, where the meetings had taken place and the extent to which full information about users' and carers' views about their involvement, problems and needs, and goals had been recorded. The aim, as in the pilot area, was to provide information for practice development. We also required the names of users eligible for care programmes, that is, who met the agreed criteria, as well as those who had actually received care programmes, in order to conduct the surveys described in the next chapters.

It has to be said that we experienced enormous difficulty in obtaining this information. For example, in one area it took six months to obtain a list of users. There appeared to be a number of reasons for this:

- There was no adequate database or CPA register. In two areas a database had been established and was being maintained. However, it emerged that this was actually a list of eligible users admitted to hospital as noted by Medical Records. There was no record of whether or not these users had actually received a care programme.

- There were genuine concerns about the confidentiality of the material. It took some time to reassure staff on this issue.

- Relatively few care programmes had actually been completed, but it was not in the interests of either the practitioners or the team managers for this fact to be known. In one area an inflated figure had been given in reports to senior managers who had been compiling returns for the DoH. (Around this time, the DoH insisted that the CPA had to be "fully implemented" within all trusts and put pressure on managers to provide confirmatory information.) This would seem to be an example of 'defensive practice'.

- Team members had been under considerable pressure and had not seen participation in audit or research as a priority.

- Some staff did not see the need for changing their practice and considered that they were "doing it all already". In particular, they did not see the need to use the CPA forms which they considered cumbersome. Others may have been privately cynical about the whole Approach and/or suffering from 'burnout'. (Onyett, Pillinger and Muijen [1995] found high levels of emotional exhaustion among nurses, social workers, psychologists and psychiatrists working in community mental health teams.)

Management action

These difficulties were conveyed to senior managers via the project advisory group meetings. To their credit, the managers acted on this information and the new area directors of the trust have secured a formal agreement with the area director of social services for the full implementation of the tiered approach. A joint agency area-wide computerised database was established. Finally, the trust selected the CPA as one of the major topics for multidisciplinary audit for the subsequent year. The clinical audit coordinator consulted us in order to define standards on user and carer involvement which are being used to construct audit criteria indicators.

What did the professionals think?

We sought the views of hospital nurses with key worker responsibilities, community psychiatric nurses and social workers, and their managers. Fifty-five staff completed questionnaires following the training sessions. Six months later, after they had experienced putting the CPA into action, we were able to follow up 30 of these staff. (By this time, four staff had left, and one was on long-term sick leave, making a response rate of 60%.) They were about equally divided between hospital and community-based staff.

Benefits of the approach

Following the training sessions, 90% of staff were positive about effect of the CPA on assessing and monitoring users' needs. At follow-up this had reduced slightly, but over 80% remained positive. They identified continuity of care as a clear benefit and observed that the CPA formalises care arrangements by providing a single, unified approach. For example:

> "The opportunity of offering the most appropriate, monitored aftercare to suit each individual."

> "Offers effective, holistic, specialised and prioritised care ... continuity of care ... maintenance of appropriate contact."

> "Collaborative interdisciplinary planning leading to clearer task allocation and improved communication between workers and clients."

One member of staff gave an impressive list of benefits:

> "... more effective assessment of client's problems, needs and capabilities ... more realistic/feasible monitoring of client's problems/needs ... promotes better quality of service - more efficient ... service delivery is enhanced ... clients involved in own care, empowering them to make constructive criticism of care and make decisions ... all appropriate agencies working effectively as a team

and communication enriched ... allows evaluation of care ... appears to be lessening readmission rate."

Disadvantages

On the other hand, it was clear that there were disadvantages. At follow-up, there was a significant increase in the number of professionals, up from 20% to 50%, commenting that the process was very time consuming, particularly in arranging meetings and filling in forms. Two thirds had anticipated that the introduction of the CPA would have a negative effect on staff workloads and administration/bureaucracy within the team and this had risen to three quarters on follow-up.

> "... more paperwork and admin means less time for actually delivering care."

One third of staff complained about procedural problems, for example, that they were not clear or too complicated or that some colleagues were opting out of their responsibilities. Multidisciplinary team working was clearly an issue, for example:

> "It is very difficult to communicate at an interdisciplinary level let alone a multidisciplinary level. It appears that some individuals are hoping CPA will 'evaporate' and they therefore aren't willing to cooperate fully in a multidisciplinary team."

Problems were thought to be both ideological,

> "There are too many differing social/medical paradigms for meaningful collaboration to happen. So that not all disciplines operate the same system with equal energy, particularly doctors."

and practical,

> "Multidisciplinary teamwork is not working because health and social services are often in conflict over eligibility criteria. There are differences in training and attitudes to client needs, often without flexibility."

However, this was a minority view - well over half the professionals considered that the CPA had had a beneficial effect on multidisciplinary team working.

Involving users

A large majority (87%) considered that the CPA had a positive effect on users' involvement in their own care, for example,

> "The input is appreciated and all work together to improve identification of requirements."

However, some reservations were expressed:

> "Clients feel pressurised and confused with CP and feel perhaps that they must comply with it when they don't want to."

> "It needs to be more flexible because some clients find CPA forms and information on them upsetting (ie, have to sign them) or threatening (eg, can't understand due to psychological disturbance)."

Surprisingly, at follow-up the professionals were equally divided in their opinions about whether the CPA would have a positive effect on users' quality of life.

> "This depends on whether they appreciate the input being provided or whether they regard it as an intrusion."

> "Positive for some clients. For certain clients, however, it focuses attention on lack of resources available to staff to improve quality of life."

Involving carers

Following the initial training, over 90% of staff anticipated that the CPA would have a positive impact on carers' involvement in the user's care. However, at follow-up this had significantly reduced to 61%, with 36% considering it had had no effect. One person commented that:

"This [carer involvement] is often in conflict with the professionals' opinions of what the client needs/is best."

But another argued,

"It makes the community mental health team more aware of influence of carers, be it positive or negative."

Disagreements

Interestingly, over three quarters of professionals had anticipated that there would be at least some disagreements between those involved in care programming: users, carers and professionals. However, at follow-up, less that half reported disagreements*. (Statistically significant differences are highlighted thus: *.) Comments included:

"In my experience discussions do not get to that point."

" ... disagreement is healthy by and large, ie, it stimulates discussion/individual views."

Personal views

At follow-up, nearly half the staff said they were satisfied with their role in care programming. However, just over half were unsure or dissatisfied. These results were not significantly different from those immediately following the training. Comments illustrate professionals' mixed feelings:

"I am pleased to say that so far my role in CPA is fine. That has only become clear after several experiences."

"[quite unsatisfied] ... I feel so frustrated, continually spending literally hours of time trying to arrange CPs at a multidisciplinary level and then being criticised for spending too much time on administration duties. This leads to feelings of powerlessness and eventually to a loss of job satisfaction."

At follow-up, 80% felt that it had been very difficult or quite difficult to implement the CPA within existing resources. For example:

"A great many decisions have to be modified to suit the resources available rather than the need of the individual."

On the other hand, another remarked:

"It's not only resources, it's attitudes, habits and beliefs and people's unwillingness to accept a different way of working...."

Many comments revealed a commitment to CPA in theory, which had been frustrated by factors such as poor management:

"I personally believe care programming to be a good, sensible concept. However, it can only work well when staff understand the concepts and are motivated and encouraged by their managers to see the benefits...."

"I am enthusiastic about CPA but my actual experience has been very negative. This should change but, with such poor health management with minuscule commitment, I feel doubtful."

"CPA is the way of the future and should be viewed positively. However, the clinging on to old ways is difficult to let go for many people. This needs to be addressed."

Summary
Positive findings

- At least 80% of staff were positive about the effects of the CPA on assessing and monitoring users' needs.

- A similar proportion considered that had a positive effect on users' involvement with their own care.

- Most thought that it had a positive impact on involving carers.

- Over half thought it benefited multidisciplinary team working.

- Many staff were strongly committed to the philosophy of the approach.

> ### *Negative findings*
>
> - Up to half said that it was very time consuming.
>
> - A third identified procedural problems.
>
> - After six months, the number of staff seeing benefits in carer involvement had dropped by a third.
>
> - 80% reported that it was difficult or very difficult to implement the CPA with existing resources.

General practitioners' views

GPs are seen by the DoH to have an important role to play in the CPA (DoH, 1995, sec 2.3). GP fundholders are expected to ensure its implementation through contracts with health trusts and specialist mental health services are advised to involve GPs in the development of individual care programmes for their patients. As part of a study we investigated the views of GPs on the principles and procedures for the CPA using a specially designed questionnaire which was sent out to all GPs in the area (Sbaraini and Carpenter, 1996b).

GPs' estimates of the percentage of adult patients with severe/long-term mental health problems on their lists ranged from none to 20%; the modal figure was 2%. Less than half the 47 respondents (34% response rate) had any experience in psychiatry, however, nearly three quarters felt able to identify patients who would benefit from specialist mental health care 'before they reached crisis point'. Fifty-one per cent "strongly agreed" that community care had placed an extra burden on their practices and a further 42% agreed.

Only one half believed they knew what a care programme was and 90% had not attended either a care programme planning or a review meeting. However, over 60% said they would be willing to attend such meetings if they had time and/or were paid. Almost all GPs stated that they wished to receive copies of the care programmes and review documents. Most (57%) supported the principle of involving users in developing care programmes, but a quarter were neutral and 15%

disagreed. They were more supportive of family carer involvement, with 72% agreeing or strongly agreeing that carers should always be involved and only 7% disagreeing.

The great majority of GPs felt that 'complex' (multidisciplinary) care programmes should be provided for patients on the Supervision Register, those leaving hospital after compulsory admission, and those having been in hospital twice or more in the previous five years. Most GPs felt a simple care programme would be most appropriate for patients leaving hospital following voluntary admission, those being admitted to hospital from, or being discharged to, residential care, and those being referred to any of the mental health services. These views were reported to the trust and have been incorporated in the development of a 'tiered system' of the CPA.

6

Evaluating users' and carers' experiences

In order to evaluate the Approach, we went back to the original set of criteria for user and carer involvement in care programming which had been worked out by the stakeholders' group (see Boxes 1 and 2). Together with the user representatives, we constructed a set of questions to assess the extent to which users, and carers, felt they had been involved in working with professionals (Box 8). (For further details of the questionnaire/interview schedule, see Appendix A.) We included a further series of questions for completion for those with care programmes, to find out what they thought about the care programmes themselves (Box 9). We also constructed a similar questionnaire for carers.

The questionnaires were coded and posted by the voluntary services office of the trust and sent to all users who, according to Medical Records, met the eligibility criteria for a care programme. The researchers did not, therefore, know the identity of respondents to the postal questionnaire. With the questionnaire was a letter explaining the purpose of the study. We were also interested in more detailed opinions and information and therefore also offered users the opportunity to be interviewed by a user or carer interviewer, for a small fee (£5).

Box 8: Questions for all users

- Are you treated with respect?
- Relationship with care manager.
- Have you been asked for your views?
- Have you been encouraged to say what your problems and needs are?
- Have you been encouraged to say what your aims are?
- Do you feel you have a choice?
- Do you feel you have a say in planning your care?
- Do you agree with your carers and the professionals?
- Information about medication, rights and services.
- Dissatisfaction and complaints.

> ## Box 9: Additional questions for users with care programmes
>
> - Did you choose to have a care programme?
> - Were you asked about the involvement of your carers?
> - Does the care programme address your needs?
> - Was it clear and comprehensive?
> - Did you agree with it?
> - How has your care programme worked out?

We also wanted to know how the care programmes had worked out. Consequently, with their agreement, we went back to the users and carers six months after the original interview or questionnaire had been completed. Although the information was not collected all at the same time (we worked on an area by area basis as the CPA was implemented across the district), we refer to Survey One as the time in each area shortly after the introduction of the CPA and Survey Two as the time six months later.

In order to get an even fuller picture of what had happened to individual service users and to try to assess the impact of the care programme on the quality of their lives using validated measures, we studied a small number of service users in depth. (We had originally hoped that the care managers would agree to use the assessment measures with their clients, with the researcher conducting follow-up evaluations. This would have given us a larger sample, but unfortunately in spite of our best effort to teach the methods and to persuade staff of the advantages, to users as well as themselves, only one social worker actually used them.) We report these as a series of case studies in Chapter 10.

Peer interviewing
Three users and a carer agreed to pilot the questionnaires by interviewing users who had a care programme and their carers. We thought that users and carers were more likely to be open and honest in discussion with other users than with professionals or researchers. We also felt that people with similar experiences to users or carers might make sympathetic interviewers, able to create an empathetic relationship with interviewees.

'Peer interviewing' is not widely used in research; it has, however, been central to this project. The pilot interviews were successful and we saw them as a positive way of ensuring continuing user and carer involvement in the evaluation. We paid the interviewers for this work and also paid the interviewees as a token of appreciation of their involvement in the research.

User and carer interviewers were recruited through forum meetings, local voluntary organisations and personal contact. They were invited to find out about the project and peer interviewing through a series of training workshops. At the workshops, one of us described the project and the interviewing process and procedures. The trainees then took part in group activities designed to facilitate discussion of important issues. This element of the workshops was important as it allowed potential interviewers to assess whether or not they wanted to take on the task. Key issues identified included: coping with interviewees' distress, confidentiality, safety, interview techniques, and procedures for arranging interviews (see Appendix A for a list and description of the materials used in training and interviewing).

After the first round of interviews was completed we held a feedback session to gain some insights into the process and to identify advantages and disadvantages. Interviewers had highlighted a number of problems, such as being paid for interviewing while claiming benefits and interviewing in interviewees' own homes. The project policy was to interview in a public place but some interviewees were agoraphobic, disabled, cared for young children, or had no transport, making this difficult. Some interviewers discovered that they knew their interviewees and, although some found this an advantage, it sometimes inhibited interviewees' openness. Interviewers also suggested improvements for training, preparation and support, such as the use of role-playing in the workshops and regular feedback/support sessions.

Interviewers' comments on their experience of peer interviewing included:

> "It's not them and us anymore."

> "She [the interviewee] said she was glad to be interviewed by me [another user]."

"I didn't mention it explicitly but there was an unspoken understanding."

Interviewers identified clear advantages of peer interviewing: breaking down the 'us and them' barrier, enhancing rapport, and, on a wider level, being involved in and making a significant contribution to a project relevant to their own personal experiences, past and present.

Across Surveys One and Two, 78 user interviews were completed (35 by users, 27 by carers and 16 by a researcher) and 15 using the carer questionnaire (13 by carers, one by a user and one by a researcher). In one area users who chose to be interviewed were given the choice of a user or a researcher. Approximately one third said they preferred a researcher. Some of the reasons given were that they would prefer to talk to a 'professional'; they feared they might meet a peer interviewer again in a difficult situation (ie, hospital); they might upset the interviewer; and that the interviewer might not keep what they had said confidential.

Overall, peer interviewing was very successful. Reassuringly, all interviewers felt able to 'contain' what was said to them in the interviews and none felt the interviewers acted inappropriately. Although interviewees were not followed up, we did give them instructions in the invitation letter on how to complain, but none contacted the research team. Interviewers generally reported that they enjoyed the interviews. The views and experiences they gathered have been combined with the answers to the confidential questionnaires to provide the project data. Information gathered in the face-to-face interviews has also been invaluable in elaborating the findings with verbatim comments and case illustrations.

The users

Overall, 109 users with severe and/or long-term mental health problems completed questionnaires or were interviewed for Survey One. Most were middle-aged, with over one third between 41 and 50 years. There were roughly equal numbers of men and women. Only 10 users had never been in hospital, whereas 60 had been admitted four times or more. Well over half the users had been sectioned (admitted to hospital involuntarily) at least once. The majority of users had been involved with services for over 10 years, with over one quarter having been involved for 20 years or more.

To summarise, the users surveyed were experienced recipients of both community and inpatient services. They were all currently on the caseloads of members of the community mental health teams. According to the local guidelines, they were all eligible for a care programme but, because the Approach was being introduced gradually, at the time of the first survey, 51 (47%) had a care programme and 58 (53%) did not. This allows us to compare the views and experiences of people with and without a care programme.

Nearly half the users (48%) lived alone, 22% lived with a partner, 20% lived in care homes and the remainder lived with relatives or friends. The only statistically significant difference between users with a care programme and those without was that users with a care programme were more likely to have been sectioned a greater number of times.

7

What the users thought - Survey One

Views of all users
Their care managers

A key principle of the CPA is that a member of the community mental health team is identified and assigned to each person in contact with services. This professional then acts as the users' first point of contact and coordinator of their care and treatment. This relationship was identified as an important one for users. Did users know who this professional was and how did they feel about him or her?

Three quarters of users said they knew who their care manager was (service users with a care programme were more likely to know this*). (There were no significant differences in the responses of users who had been interviewed and those who had completed questionnaires; we have therefore combined the results.) Some users clearly had a care manager but were not familiar with the jargon, as this quotation illustrates:

> "I see a social worker and a CPN but I don't know who the care manager is."

The vast majority of users were *very positive* about their care manager: nearly 90% felt *comfortable* with their care manager and felt that they *treated them with respect.* Typical comments included:

> "I'm very happy with my care manager. I like to talk things through with her."

> "I feel I am treated with respect."

> "I'm working together with my CPN."

Users' positive responses reflect the fact that regular contact with one professional facilitated the development of a stable, trusting relationship, enhancing service delivery and continuity of care.

The majority of users said they did not mind if their care manager was male or female (59%). However, nearly one third (32%) expressed a preference for a woman and 9% preferred a man. Women were more likely to express a preference, while both men and women tended to prefer a care manager of the same gender*.

Choice and involvement in services

One of the central aims of the evaluation was to investigate the extent to which users *feel involved in their own mental health care* and to see whether or not having a care programme effects this. Table 1 shows how all the users surveyed responded to a number of questions designed to investigate this issue. Responses given by users with a care programme and those without, which show clear *differences* in their opinions, are given in Table 2.

Table 1: Involvement: views of all users (%)

	Yes	No	Unsure
Have you been asked what you thought about your admission to hospital and/or involvement with services?	31	60	9
Do you feel you have been encouraged by professionals to say what your aims are for care and treatment?	63	31	6
Do you feel you have a choice in your care and treatment when in hospital?	32	59	9
Do you feel you have a choice in your care and treatment when in the community?	76	22	2

Table 1 shows that less than one third of users felt they had been asked their opinions on being admitted to hospital and/or being involved with services. However, nearly two thirds felt encouraged by professionals to talk about their aims for their care and treatment. These findings may reflect the fact that professionals felt more at ease or found it more relevant to talk to users about their future care and treatment, rather than their experiences in hospital or their feelings about being involved with services at all. However, in the stakeholder discussions, users identified being asked about hospital admission and/or referral to services as important for their sense of involvement.

Not surprisingly, users felt that they had more choice in their care and treatment when in the community than in hospital*.

Table 2: Involvement: views of users with and without a care programme (%)

	Yes		No		Unsure	
	CP	No CP	CP	No CP	CP	No CP
Do you feel able to work out a plan with professionals for your care and treatment?	84	61	14	28	2	11
Do you feel you have a choice in your care and treatment when in the community?	86	68	14	28	0	4
Have you been encouraged by professionals to say what your problems and needs are?	74	60	16	38	10	2
Do you feel you have a say in planning your care?	69	55	27	43	4	2

Note: CP = care programme

Table 2 shows that both users with a care programme and those without gave a greater number of positive rather than negative responses. However, users with a care programme gave *more* positive responses than those without a care programme. They felt more able to work with professionals* and say what their problems and needs were*, they felt they had more choice in their care and treatment in the community* and they felt they had more say in planning their mental health care*. *These findings show the positive effect of having a care programme on users' feelings of involvement and choice.*

Problems and needs

Users in the stakeholder discussions identified being able to state their own views about their problems and needs (not to have them solely 'diagnosed' by others) as important in encouraging their sense of involvement. Table 2 shows that the majority of users felt able to do this (and users with a care programme felt more able*). We also wanted to find out if users tended to agree or disagree with the following people about their problems and needs (see Table 3).

Table 3: Problems and needs

	Agree	Disagree	Unsure
Carer	55 (80%)	5 (7%)	9 (13%)
Care manager	56 (74%)	9 (12%)	11 (14%)
Psychiatrist	46 (52%)	28 (32%)	14 (16%)
Family	33 (44%)	28 (38%)	13 (18%)

Overall, users were more likely to agree, than disagree, with the people listed. However, users were much more likely to agree with their (non-family) carer and care manager than their psychiatrist* or family*. The finding that three quarters or more of the users surveyed tended to agree with their care manager and carer is encouraging as these are the people likely to be most closely involved in the planning and delivery of their care.

However, approximately one in three users disagreed with their psychiatrist and family about their problems and needs (although quite a few gave the 'unsure' response). A number of users commented on the poor communication they had with their psychiatrist:

> "I disagreed with the psychiatrist about being labelled schizophrenic ... we haven't talked since!"

> " ... dreadful communication with the psychiatrist ... we don't actually disagree because he never even answers a question."

Although many users wanted a carer (usually a relative) involved in their care, some commented that their family had contributed to their problems or they were not supportive:

> "My family are the main problem and the influence they have over me."

> "My family have always been negative."

Medication

In the stakeholders' discussions of involvement and empowerment, medication had been identified as an important part of many users' lives. It was agreed that users needed to be fully informed about their medication - its nature, purpose, side-effects and any alternatives. The Patients' Charter also states that, in order to give *informed* consent to a treatment, the recipient must be told about these things. The vast majority of users surveyed (nearly 90%) were taking medication for psychiatric symptoms, making information provision an important issue.

Figure 1 shows that users were more likely to have been informed about the nature and purpose of their medication than have been told about possible side-effects* or alternatives and their right to refuse it*. In other words, users were more likely to be told positive things about their medication (ie, how it would help) rather than anything that might 'put them off' taking it (ie, possible side-effects).

Reassuringly, 79% of users said their medication was reviewed regularly and 81% of these said that reviews were at intervals of less than three months.

Figure 1: "Have you been told about ...?"

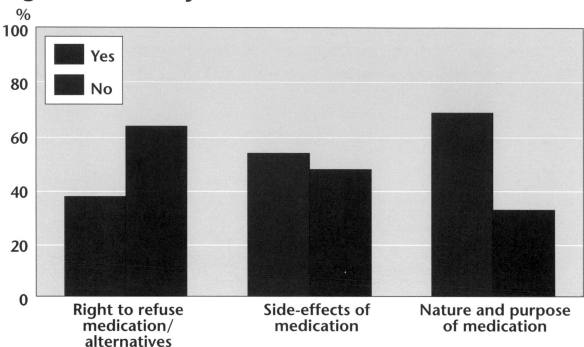

Complaints

It is important that both users and carers feel able to express dissatisfaction or complain about any aspect of care they disagree with. This ability implies that they feel confident in dealing with services and means that services are better able to identify any problems and improve quality on a continual basis.

Seventy per cent of users said they would feel able to say if they were dissatisfied about an aspect of their care. However, a smaller portion, 57%, said they would feel able to make a complaint. This implies that users felt more at ease expressing their dissatisfaction informally. Comments on what inhibited users to complain included:

> "I would feel able to put in a complaint but only if I was well at the time."

> "I would be frightened to complain."

> "I have complained by have not been listened to."

> "If I did complain they might put me away again."

Half the users surveyed had *thought about making a complaint* and only just over half were aware that the health authority and social services have official complaints procedures (users with a care programme were more likely to be aware of this*). These are disturbing findings and highlight the need for users to feel empowered to be able to complain, as well as be properly informed about complaints procedures.

Summary
Positive findings
- The vast majority of users were very positive about their relationship with their care manager.

- The majority of users felt encouraged by professionals to say what their aims were for their care and treatment and to say what their problems and needs were; they felt they had a choice in their care and treatment when in the community; and they felt able to work out a plan with professionals for their care and treatment.

- Approximately three out of four users were in agreement with both their carers and care managers about their problems and needs.

Negative findings
- Some service users had not given their informed consent to medication treatment.

- A significant proportion of users had not been asked what they thought about their admission to hospital and/or involvement with services; felt they had little a choice in their care and treatment when in hospital; and did not feel they had a say in planning their care.

- Nearly one third of users disagreed with their psychiatrist about their problems and needs.

- Half the users had thought about making a complaint about their care and treatment and just less than half did not know that official complaints procedures existed.

Users with care programmes

Users with care programmes were asked a further series of questions about the process of care programming and about the care programmes themselves.

Carer involvement

One of the key principles of the CPA is to involve carers in users' care planning. Table 4 shows who users specified as their main carer.

Over one quarter of users did not specify a carer and 20% specified a member of one of the community mental health teams. Another 17 users named a different professional (ie, care staff, GP) while the remaining 42 named a relative or friend. We were interested in the views and experiences of the 59 users (54%) whose carers were not a member of the community mental health team.

Table 4: Main carers		
Main carer		
Member of the community mental health team	22	(20%)
Partner	21	(19%)
Residential care staff	14	(13%)
Parent	14	(13%)
Friend	4	(3%)
GP/psychiatrist	3	(3%)
Son/daughter	2	(2%)
Sister/brother	1	(1%)
No one specified/missing	28	(26%)
Total	109	(100%)

Nearly three quarters of these users *wanted their carer involved* in their care. It is perhaps surprising that one in four users did not want or were unsure about the person they saw as their main carer being involved in their care planning. Comments included:

"I want my husband involved because he knows me and lives with me."

"I feel as if I don't want to bother anyone about my own problems."

"I would get more support from my family if they were involved ... the more they know, the easier it would be for them to understand."

Over 70% of users felt their carers *discussed their care/treatment with professionals.* Users with a care programme were more likely to report this*. It is important to recognise that a minority of users were happy that their carers were not consulted.

Figure 2: "Have you been asked if you want your carer involved in planning your care?"

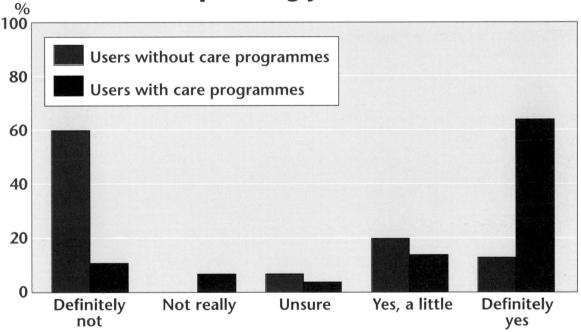

The majority (58%) of users felt their *carers views were listened* to the *right amount.* However, 22% felt they *weren't listened to enough,* 13% felt they were listened to *too much* and 6% felt they were not listened to at all (although some users were happy with this situation).

Carers should be asked if they *want a carer involved in their care planning* as part of the CPA process. Figure 2 illustrates that users with a care programme were much more likely to have been asked*.

Rights and services

It is important that users and carers are well informed about mental health services, both statutory and voluntary. Only if users and carers have adequate information about rights and services will they be able to get the most out of them. Table 5 shows how many users overall, and with and without a care programme, reported that they had received information on a variety of relevant subjects.

Table 5: "Have you been given information about ...?" (%)

	Total - Yes	Care programme - Yes	No care programme - Yes
How to get benefits advice*	60	71	50
Access to community mental health services*	50	65	36
Right to see medical records	42	49	36
Local user forums	35	37	33
Right not to have a care programme*	35	57	16
Rights with respect to the Mental Health Act - if sectioned*	33	45	22
Citizen Advocacy Service*	28	41	17
Out of hours services*	28	39	17

Service users with a care programme were more likely to have been given information on *six out of the eight rights and services* listed than those without (the eight rights and services were listed in the original care programme forms for discussion with the user). For only two of the rights and services listed were half or more of all the users provided with information. Clearly, users need to be better informed about relevant rights and services. However, it should be noted that local user forums, the Citizens Advocacy Service and out of hours services were not fully established in all areas at the time of the research. Also, rights with regard to the Mental Health Act would only apply to users who had been sectioned.

Summary
Differences between users with a care programme and those without
Users with a care programme were more likely to:

- know who their care manager was
- feel they had more choice in their care and treatment in the community
- feel they had a say in planning their mental health care
- feel encouraged by professionals to say what their problem and needs were
- feel able to take an active part in working out a plan with professionals for their care and treatment
- have been asked if they wanted a carer involved in planning their care
- report that their carer discussed their care and treatment with mental health workers
- have been given information about rights and services.

What did they think of their care programmes?

As well as gathering all the users' experiences and views of different aspects of services, users with care programmes were asked specific questions about them. These questions were developed during the stakeholders' discussions and included some of a practical nature (ie, did users have a copy of their care programmes? were they asked to sign them?) and others designed to evaluate the care programmes (did users feel their needs were addressed? were their care programmes clear and comprehensive?).

Of the 51 users who had a care programme, nearly three quarters said that they had a copy. Of the one quarter who did not have a copy, 64% said that they would have liked one. Over three quarters of users said they had signed their care programme. Only one user said that they could not remember the initial care programme meeting. Figure 3 shows where the care programme meetings took place.

Figure 3: Venue of initial care programme meetings

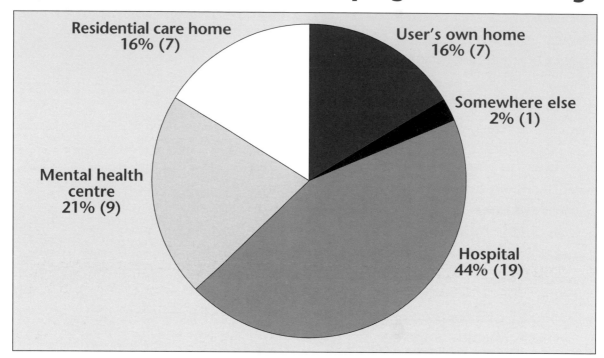

Residential care home
16% (7)

User's own home
16% (7)

Somewhere else
2% (1)

Mental health
centre
21% (9)

Hospital
44% (19)

Sixty-two per cent of users said their care programme had already been reviewed. Of those users who said that their care programme had not been reviewed, approximately one third said a review was planned, one third were unsure and one third said that one wasn't planned.

Figure 4 shows users' evaluations of various aspects of their care programme.

Users were generally positive about their care programmes. Over three quarters felt they were clear and comprehensive, agreed with them and felt they addressed their needs. Fewer users felt they had worked out well, although a large proportion were unsure (many commented that it was too early to say). Although the majority of users felt able to choose whether or not to have a care programme, a substantial minority felt they didn't or were unsure. Some commented that they were simply told they had to have one or they thought having a care programme was just part of their statutory care arrangements. More detailed care programme evaluations are given in the case profiles, Chapter 10.

Figure 4: Care programme evaluation

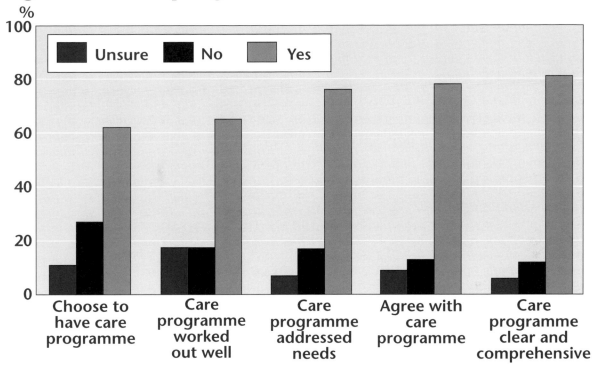

8
What the carers thought

The carers

Carers were asked if they would like to take part in the research through our contact with the user, that is, when the user completed a questionnaire or was interviewed they were asked if they would mind their carer taking part. This meant that carers only took part in the research with their own and the user's agreement. (From this point on the person the carer provides care for will be referred to as their 'relative', even though not all carers were related to the person they cared for.)

Twenty carers completed questionnaires or were interviewed. There were 11 men and 9 women. Eleven carers were providing care/support to a relative with a care programme and nine were giving care/support to a relative without a care programme.

Half the carers surveyed were partners (10) and one third were parents (7). One was a friend and two were residential care staff. The majority of carers were between the ages of 30 and 50 years. Two thirds of carers had been involved with services for up to 10 years and the remaining third had been involved for 11 years or more.

To summarise, most carers were related to the user, were middle-aged and were experienced in dealing with services.

Carers' views
Involvement in relatives' care

In the stakeholder discussions carers, like users, stressed that their participation in their relatives' care also needed to be actively encouraged by professionals. Carers were asked the same four questions about their involvement as their relatives. Ninety-five per cent of carers said that *they wanted to be involved in their relatives' care* and 5% were unsure. *None of the carers said that they did not want to be involved in their relatives' care.* Carers gave various reasons for wanting to be involved in planning their relatives' care:

"So as to understand the mental health service better."

"... because it affects me and my children."

"I have loads of questions I'd like to ask."

Two thirds of carers felt they *discussed their relatives' care/treatment with professionals,* although one third said they didn't. One added:

"The CPN can only do what he is allowed to do in the time available."

An equal number of carers felt that their views were and were *not listened to by professionals* (8, 40%), and nearly a quarter (4, 20%) were unsure. Carers highlighted a discrepancy between *discussing* their relatives' care and treatment with professionals and actually being *listened to.*

Just over half (53%) the carers felt that they had not been asked if they wanted to be involved in their relatives' care. Carers whose relatives had a care programme were much more likely to report that they had been asked*. One carer whose relative had a care programme said he had definitely been asked:

"... by the social worker."

Another carer whose relative did not have a care programme and who felt that he had not been asked added:

"The professionals seemed to make up their minds on what was to happen and I was told afterwards."

It is disappointing that over half the carers felt they had not been asked if they wanted to be involved in their relatives' care. As the above quotation illustrates, some carers felt totally excluded from the process of making care arrangements. Others also commented that their needs were ignored:

"There's no support for me and the kids. They suffer too - it effects the whole family."

Care managers

In order for carers to play an active part in planning their relatives' mental healthcare with professionals, it is clearly important for them to be familiar with and have a good relationship with their relative's care manager.

The majority of carers (70%) said they knew who their relative's care manager was. Some carers were not familiar with these professionals because their relatives were not in regular contact with a member of the community mental health team. Carers whose relatives had a care programme were more likely to know who the case manager was*.

All the carers who were familiar with their relative's care manager said that they felt these professionals treated them (the carers) with *respect* and 90% of carers felt *comfortable* with the care manager.

Like their relatives, carers were generally very positive about the care manager and appreciated the development of a stable, trusting, one-to one relationship with a professional. Typical comments included:

"The CPN has built up a good relationship with both of us."

"Good rapport with present care manager."

Choice and involvement in services

Carers were asked the same questions as their relatives to explore the degree to which they felt involved with services (see Table 6).

The majority of carers responded positively to most of the questions. Two thirds reported that they had been asked their opinions on their relative's hospital admission and/or involvement with mental health services. One commented:

"It has been discussed with me during the last two years."

but another added:

"I've been asked but my comments were not taken into consideration."

Table 6: Involvement: views of all carers (%)

	Yes	No	Unsure
Have you been asked what you thought about your relative's admission to hospital and/or involvement with services?	**65**	**35**	0
Do you feel you have been encouraged by professionals to say what your aims are for your relative's care and treatment?	**60**	35	5
Do you feel your relative has a choice in their care and treatment when in hospital?	**60**	37	13
Do you feel your relative has a choice in their care and treatment when in the community?	**88**	6	6
Do you feel able to work out a plan with professionals for your relative's care and treatment?	**84**	16	0
Have you been encouraged by professionals to say what your views are about your relative's problems and needs?	45	**55**	0
Do you feel you have a say in planning your relative's care?	**53**	42	5

Sixty per cent of carers felt encouraged to say what their aims were for their relatives' care and treatment. However, this means that over one third did not really feel encouraged to express their views.

Like their relatives, carers felt there was more choice in care and treatment in the community, rather than in hospital.

The majority of carers felt able to work out a plan with professionals for their relatives' care and treatment. One carer whose relative had a care programme commented that he felt able to do this because:

"We have a meeting once a month. Everything is discussed and sorted out thoroughly."

Others commented:

"I would feel very able to take an active part in working out a plan but getting my relative to agree would be extremely difficult."

"Professionals do not usually make contact."

On the less positive side, less than half the carers felt encouraged to state their views on their relatives' problems and needs. Comments included:

"... professionals don't take any notice of me."

"I feel the care manager does her best but her case-load is heavy - she is always busy so there is not always the opportunity."

Overall, just over half the carers felt they had a say in planning their relative's mental healthcare, although a substantial minority (42%) felt they didn't. Two unhappy carers whose relatives did not have care programmes commented:

"No one has ever approached me to ask my opinions."

and:

"I can never plan my own life because I am always having to take my son's needs into consideration."

The mixed responses show that, while some professionals were very successful in encouraging carers to state their views and be involved in their relative's care, others had not.

Comments on what carers *liked best* about services included:

"The groups my wife goes to twice a week and the help from the mental health worker."

"They take account of my wife's needs and what she feels comfortable with."

"Constant help from psychiatrist, mental health workers and therapy."

and what they *liked least:*

"No help provided for me."

"Not being able to get anything done at the weekends if my spouse breaks down."

"The length of time to sort things out, the lack of contact and the feeling that the medics are fumbling in the dark."

"The difficulties caused by funding."

Problems and needs

Carers, like their relatives, were asked if they tended to agree or disagree with the following people about their relatives' problems and needs:

Table 7: Problems and needs

	Agree	Disagree	Unsure
Psychiatrist	10 (84%)	1 (8%)	1 (8%)
Relative	11 (69%)	3 (19%)	2 (12%)
Care manager	9 (64%)	3 (22%)	2 (14%)
Family	6 (50%)	2 (17%)	4 (33%)

The majority of carers tended to agree, rather than disagree, with the people listed. Carers were most likely to agree with the psychiatrist, followed by their relative, and least likely to agree with other members of the family (although one third of carers gave an 'unsure' response when asked about family - this question may have been irrelevant in some cases). Although the numbers are small, it is encouraging to see that less than one quarter of carers disagreed with the people listed and the majority were in agreement with their relative.

Medication

Voluntary organisations, such as the National Schizophrenia Fellowship, have argued that, if carers are to play a part in supporting service users, then they must be well informed about the user's treatments. This includes information about medication. Carers were asked the same questions as their relatives about medication.

Just over half the carers were aware of their relative's right to refuse medication and be told of alternatives. Half were informed of the side-effects, but the majority had not been told how the medication worked or should help their relative. Carers would clearly benefit from being more informed about their relative's medication. However, it is possible that some service users didn't want their carers to know about it. 16 (80%) carers said that their relative's medication was reviewed regularly, although some commented that they would like it to be reviewed more frequently, that is, every three months rather than every six months.

Complaints

Three quarters of carers said they would be able to say if they were *dissatisfied* with any aspect of their relative's care and 85% said they would feel reasonably *able to complain* if they needed to. Carers reported feeling more able to express dissatisfaction and complain than their relatives. Fear of repercussions due to making a complaint expressed by users (ie, services being withdrawn or imposed) was probably less significant for carers.

Just over a third of carers said they had *thought about complaining* about their relative's care and treatment. Nearly three quarters said they were aware that the health authority and social services have official complaints procedures. When compared to their relatives, carers were less likely to have thought about complaining and more likely to know about official complaints procedures. One carer commented:

"We went to the GP and social worker who changed the psychiatrist."

One carer, whose husband did not have a care programme, said she had thought about complaining about:

"The social worker's interference."

To summarise, the majority of carers surveyed were informed about complaints procedures and felt able to express dissatisfaction or make a complaint. However, some expressed doubt as to whether or not this would be a helpful move or would make any difference:

"I don't like stirring things up as it seems to be detrimental rather than being extra help."

Rights and services

Carers were asked if they were informed about the same eight rights and services as their relatives. The majority of carers felt they knew how to get benefits advice. For all the other rights and services listed, the majority felt they *had not* been given information. However, carers whose relatives had a care programme were more likely to be informed about the Citizens Advocacy Service* and how to contact services out of hours*. Again, these findings highlight the lack of information being provided for those using or in contact with services.

Do carers and clients tend to agree or disagree with each other?

The responses of the carers who were surveyed were matched and compared to the responses given by their relatives. There were no major differences between their opinions, showing that, on the whole, carers and users tended to agree with each other. This is perhaps not surprising when the users surveyed said that they agreed with their carers most about their problems and needs. Although carers were most likely to agree with the psychiatrist, they were second most likely to agree with their relative. Also, the carers who took part only did so with the agreement of their relatives. Clients who disagreed with their carers or who did not want them involved in their care could have been less likely to agree to their taking part in the survey in the first place. However, it is still an important finding that users and carers tended to agree with each other and adds weight to the argument that carers should be involved as much as possible in their relative's care if both parties are in agreement.

Summary
Positive findings

- Nearly 100% of carers wanted to be involved in their relative's care.

- Two thirds of carers discussed their views on involvement with professionals.

- The majority of carers had been asked what they thought about their relative's admission to hospital and/or involvement with services; felt encouraged by professionals to say what their aims were for their relative's care and treatment; felt their relatives had choice in their care and treatment; and felt able to work out a plan with professionals for their relative's care and treatment.

- The majority of carers were informed about complaints procedures and felt able to express dissatisfaction and make a complaint.

- Carers and users tended to agree with each.

Negative findings

- One third of carers had not been asked what they thought about their relative's involvement with services and/or admission to hospital.

- Less than half the carers felt their views were listened to by professionals.

- Many carers were not adequately informed about their relative's medication.

- The majority of carers were not adequately informed about relevant rights and services.

- A significant proportion did not feel encouraged by professionals to say what their views were about their relative's problems and needs; and did not feel they had a say in planning their relative's care.

What they thought of the care programme

The 11 carers whose relatives had received care programmes were asked specific questions about them. Briefly, we found that:

- 100% felt the care programme was mostly clear and comprehensive
- 100% felt it addressed their relative's needs
- 80% felt their relative was able to choose whether or not to have one
- 80% mostly agreed with the care programme
- 70% felt the care programme had worked out well to some extent
- 70% felt the care programme had increased their relative's independence.

Positive comments included:

"I thought it was the right step to help my spouse regain the confidence lost through being ill."

"It helped my husband to socialise with people which he hadn't been able to do."

"(My wife is becoming more independent) Ö especially with the groups at the mental health centre. They have shown her how to be more assertive."

"It kept my husband occupied and gave me a breathing space."

"Ideas were taken into account and discussed with all concerned."

"I'm happy there's an agreement for my son's care and I can question things if they are not done."

and negative:

"My wife's care manager is trying to do the very best for her but, unfortunately, my concerns and observations have not been recognised. I would appreciate closer involvement in my wife's care programme."

"The CP was set up months ago and that's all I know about it."

One carer said that she was frustrated that a care programme had been worked out with her and her husband but that he had "refused to stick to it".

Summary
Differences between carers whose relatives have and do not have a care programme
Carers whose relatives had a care programme were more likely to:

- report that they had been asked if they wanted to be involved in their relative's care
- know who their relative's care manager was
- be informed about some of the rights and services listed.

9

Users' and carers' views and experiences six months later - Survey Two

Users (and carers) were 'followed up' approximately six months after they took part in Survey One. The aim was to see if their care and treatment had changed in that time and if so, did this influence their views. We were particularly interested to see how the care programmes had developed - did users feel their care programmes had delivered what had been promised or had users become disillusioned with the CPA process?

For Survey One, 109 users were interviewed or completed questionnaires. Twenty-eight users could not be included in Survey Two, leaving 81 people (19 users were not invited to take part in Survey Two because they were interviewed only a short time previously for Survey One, three users had died, two had moved out of the area, two were too ill to take part, one was in hospital and one was no longer involved in services).

A total of 44 users (54%) took part in Survey Two. Figure 5 shows how many users did and did not have care programmes at the time of Surveys One and Two.

Seventeen users had care programmes at the time of Surveys One and Two and 17 did not have care programmes at the time of both surveys. Six users who did not have care programmes at Survey One had them at Survey Two, and four users who had care programmes at Survey One did not have them at the time of Survey Two. We will now examine these four groups in more detail.

Figure 5: "Do you have a care programme?"

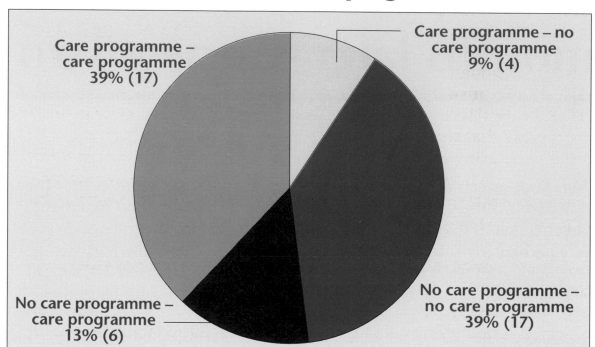

Care programme –
care programme
39% (17)

Care programme – no
care programme
9% (4)

No care programme –
care programme
13% (6)

No care programme –
no care programme
39% (17)

No care programme at Survey One - no care programme at Survey Two

Responses given in Survey Two by users who had never had a care programme were not markedly different from those given in Survey One. This would be expected - there is no reason to anticipate that these users' experiences and views of services would have changed because they would still, essentially, be experiencing the same level of support (ie, no care programme).

No care programme at Survey One - care programme at Survey Two

We would anticipate some change in the views of those six users who had had a care programme since Survey One. Although very small in number, the views of these users were generally more positive at Survey Two. For example, five out of six said they definitely had been asked if they wanted their carer involved in planning their care, were able to say what there problems and needs were and felt they had choice in the community at Survey Two. They were also better informed about rights and services.

Care programme at Survey One - no care programme at Survey Two

It is unclear why four users had care programmes at Survey One but not at Survey Two. All of these users completed questionnaires at Survey One and, although all of them said that they had care programmes, none of them answered all the questions in the care programme evaluation section of the questionnaires (two left it completely blank). It is possible that some of these users never had a care programme, perhaps confusing it with a care programme developed for hospital or a residential care home. However, two of the users had a care manager at the time of both surveys and it is possible that the care programmes had never been reviewed or that the users had forgotten about it.

Care programme at Survey One - care programme at Survey Two

Very similar differences to those in Survey One, between users with care programmes and users without, were found when looking at the Survey Two data on its own, that is, users with care programmes were more likely to know who their care manager was*; feel they had more choice in their care and treatment in the community*; have a say in planning their mental healthcare*; feel encouraged by professionals to say what their problem and needs were*; feel able to take an active part in working out a plan with professionals for their care and treatment*; have been asked if they wanted a carer involved in planning their care*; and have been given information about some rights and services*.

However, the group of most interest were those who had care programmes at the time of both Surveys. The major areas of change for these users was with the involvement of carers. Users were less likely to report that they had been asked if they wanted their carer involved in their care* and that their carer discussed their care and treatment with mental health workers* at Survey Two. However, users were also less likely to want their carers involved in their care planning* at Survey Two*. One user said that he no longer wanted his carer to be so responsible for him (see the second case profile, Donald). Other users whose care programmes had been in place for some time and whose circumstances were relatively stable may have felt that support from their carers was less necessary. There were no other marked differences in users' opinions with regard to the other areas service, such as medication, relationship with care manager and involvement in services.

As far as the care programme evaluations were concerned, although users were, on the whole, slightly less positive in their evaluations, these differences were not dramatic. However, from the in-depth interviews it became clear that not all care programmes had been progressing in a similar way. It was possible to identify and place users' evaluations into three general categories: those who were consistently positive about their care programmes across the surveys (10 users); those who were more mixed in their opinions at Survey Two (four users); and those who had become disillusioned with the CPA process by Survey Two (three users). Case examples, taken from the face-to-face interviews, have been used to illustrate these differences (see Chapter 10).

Summary of findings - carers

Eight carers were interviewed for Survey Two. Four were caring for relatives who had care programmes at Surveys One and Two, three were caring for users who had never had a care programme, and one was caring for a user who did not have a care programme at Survey One but had one at Survey Two.

Three of the four carers whose relatives had care programmes commented that they were no longer really involved with the care programmes (two did not know if their relative still had a care programme). However, one carer was very satisfied with services at the time of both surveys (see first case profile, Ruth). The carer whose relative had only recently had a care programme was much more positive about services at Survey Two.

All of the carers of relatives who did not have care programmes felt that both they and their relatives had little support. Overall, six of the eight carers expressed feelings of isolation and frustration. These carers often commented on the lack of information they had about services and community resources and expressed fears about what would happen to their relatives if they could no longer cope with caring for them (see third and fourth case profiles, Carol and Robert).

Assessing outcomes

In order to assess the outcomes of the care programmes we monitored the progress of seven users with care programmes using two measures, Goal Attainment Scaling, and a Quality of Life questionnaire.

Goal Attainment Scaling

(See Appendix A for a more detailed description of this measure.)

The seven users identified a number of personal goals in important areas of their lives and worked out Goal Attainment Scalings at Survey One. They were followed up six months later at Survey Two to find out what level of attainment they had achieved on each personal goal.

A total of 18 goals were scaled at Survey One, that is, an average of 2.5 goals by each user. Eight goals were of a practical nature (eg, to go shopping, improve budgeting, sort out benefits), six were based on improving mental health (eg, reduce anxiety, increase positive thoughts, control voices) and four were of a social nature (eg, go to social club, increase structured day time activities).

At Survey Two users had achieved the highest level of attainment for 11 goals, the middle level for three goals, the lower level for two goals and for two goals there had been no change (there had not been a deterioration in any of the goal areas).

Users' views were mixed as to whether or not their achievements had been influenced by their care programmes. Comments included:

> "Changes [reduction of depression and anxiety] have come from my own efforts."

> "My social worker has made sure I'm claiming all the benefits I'm entitled to and helps me with budgeting."

> "I found the voluntary work myself, through my local church, the mental health team didn't have anything to do with it."

> "All the help and support I've got has given me the confidence to get out and about and do my own shopping."

It is difficult to assess accurately the extent to which having a care programme contributed to users' achieving their personal goals. What is clear, however, was that users found it relatively easy to identify and scale up meaningful personal goals from the problems/needs they identified in their care programmes. Goal Attainment Scaling offered a useful way of measuring individuals' aspirations and most users were pleased to see the extent to which they had achieved these.

Quality of Life
(See Appendix A for a more detailed description of this measure.)

The same seven users also completed the Lancashire Quality of Life Scale at Surveys One and Two. This standardised interview measures allowed us to see if there had been any changes in satisfaction with different areas of their lives over time. For example, it could be anticipated that achieving a desired change in accommodation (ie, moving from a hostel to one's own flat) would be reflected by an increase in satisfaction in the 'living situation' dimension of the Quality of Life measure. Would the achievement of personal goals (as specified in individuals' Goal Attainment Scaling) be reflected in increased life satisfaction in the relevant areas?

Changes in individual Quality of Life scores are described in some of the case profiles. Looking at the group as a whole, however, there were no marked differences to the average scores given at Surveys One and Two. Examining the average Survey One scores and rounding them up, a score of five (quite satisfied) was given for five life areas (leisure, religion, living situation, social relations and health), a score of four (mixed) for four areas (general well-being, work/education, finances, and family relations) and a score of six for the 'legal and safety' area. These average scores are comparable to those given by similar user groups.

Changes in satisfaction in an individual's different life areas sometimes appeared to fit in with life changes that had occurred between Surveys One and Two, whereas others didn't (see the case profiles for examples). Achievements in Goal Attainment Scaling were often *not* reflected in increased satisfaction in the relevant life area. For example, the second case profile, Donald, shows a user who had achieved his goal of doing voluntary work but whose pleasure at this was overridden by a fear that he would never return to full-time paid employment.

10
Case profiles

These case profiles follow four users over a period of six months, three with a care programme and one without. Goal Attainment Scaling and the Lancashire Quality of Life Scale measure have been used to provide quantitative information on the effect of the care programmes. Three examples provide detailed illustrations of the diverse outcomes of the CPA process for different users, as shown in the research findings. The first illustration describes a situation in which the CPA process had been mainly successful. The second case illustrates a more mixed outcome, while the third example shows a total breakdown of the CPA process. The fourth example charts the care and treatment of an eligible user who had never had a care programme. All names used in this section have been changed.

Ruth: a success story

Ruth, a middle-aged woman living with her husband, had been involved with services for over 20 years, and had been admitted to hospital many times, sometimes under Section. She had recently been admitted to hospital due to a 'breakdown'. A care programme had been in place since her discharge. Both Ruth and her husband David were very positive about their recent experiences with services.

Ruth said that she definitely felt that she had a say in planning her mental healthcare. She had definitely been asked by professionals if she wanted a carer involved in her care and said that she did. Her husband discussed her care and treatment thoroughly with mental health workers and Ruth felt that he was listened to appropriately. Ruth saw her social worker two times a week and was happy with their relationship. She felt informed about her medication and rights and services. She felt encouraged by professionals to state her views, discussed her care and treatment thoroughly with them and concluded:

> "... since my latest release from hospital my husband and I have been very satisfied with the support and help of all the mental health workers."

Ruth's evaluation of her care programme was also very positive and she concluded that:

> "... this really feels like care in the community."

David commented that his wife's care had improved greatly since the care programme and a change of psychiatrist. Like his wife, he felt able to communicate well with professionals, felt involved in her care planning, was well informed about medication, rights and services and felt his wife's needs were being properly addressed.

Ruth was generally positive about the various aspects of her life described in the Quality of Life measure and her self-esteem was high. She identified three personal goals through Goal Attainment Scaling: to be able to shop on her own, drive on her own and to reduce the amount of time spent with a relative.

Six months later

Ruth's responses in the second interview were quite similar. When asked about her care programme, she commented:

> "I am very satisfied with it all."

When asked if the care programme addressed her needs she replied "definitely yes" but added:

> "... within the confines of the economics of the health system."

At Survey Two David also remained very positive but expressed concerns about funding and its effects on his wife's care and treatment:

> "Due to recent cut backs her care manager only visits once a week, it used to be twice."

Again, he was very satisfied with the care programme and its positive effect on his wife but was worried that support would be reduced:

> "The cut backs are a disaster for anyone with a mental health problem. I hope they don't mean a return to how my wife was before because she is so well now."

Ruth's Quality of Life had remained generally positive, her self-esteem was still high and she had achieved all of her personal aims as specified in the Goal Attainment Scaling.

Summary
Both Ruth and David felt that the care programme had been a real success and noted how much happier they were with current services. Both felt involved in the care and treatment being provided and had built up good relationships with professionals. They felt that Ruth was being fully supported, that her needs were being met and this had greatly improved her mental health. However, they expressed concern about Ruth's support from the community mental health team being reduced and the effect this might have on her mental health (although the improvement in her health would perhaps imply a decreased need for input).

Donald: a mixed outcome
Donald, in his mid-twenties and living by himself, had been diagnosed with schizophrenia 18 months ago. He had been admitted to hospital, both voluntarily and under Section, on six or seven occasions in that time and had tried seven different medications. However, he wasn't taking any medication at the time of the interview and felt he was coping much better without it. He commented:

> "It doesn't work for me. I've tried 7 and I get on much better without it. Having an injection takes away your dignity - having someone stick a needle in your bum - and it bloody hurts!"

He was very dissatisfied with the psychiatrist and community psychiatric nurse he had before his care programme. He felt that all they offered him was medication that hadn't worked (ie, reduced the voices) and had serious side-effects (ie, excessive weight gain and loss of libido). He felt they had little insight into or understanding of his situation.

Donald's initial care programme meeting was in hospital several months previously and he was given a copy of the document. He said that he had been asked if he wanted a non-professional carer involved in his care programme, to which he replied positively. He added that his carer (a parent) discussed his care and treatment thoroughly with mental health workers. His care programme had been largely developed with his new care manager, a different community psychiatric nurse, and focused on providing day activities, support and monitoring for Donald.

Donald said that he had felt encouraged by professionals to say what his problems and needs were and that he "totally agreed" with his community psychiatric nurse. However, he "totally disagreed" with his psychiatrist. He felt he had been able to work with professionals on his care programme and that he had choice in his care and treatment in the community. He commented that he was being helped to become more independent but still needed support. Donald was very positive about his current community psychiatric nurse, whom he saw once every two weeks, finding her sympathetic and supportive. He commented:

> "My CPN is brilliant."

He no longer saw a psychiatrist, but saw a psychologist with whom he was much happier. He said that he appreciated the chance to talk about what he was going through rather than being given a prescription or an injection. Donald attended and chaired a 'Hearing Voices' support group fortnightly and found the mutual support rewarding.

Donald had found resources in the community very poor and this is why he saw no point in attending them. Donald had plenty of ideas about what would improve services: properly resourced community centres with workshops, art rooms, computers with games, sports facilities, access to a mini bus to provide outings and better organised regular support groups:

> "People need to have something to do, not just sit and smoke and drink tea."

Donald's assessment of his satisfaction with various aspect of his life were generally positive. On four of out of the nine areas of life satisfaction he said that his situation "couldn't be better". However, two main areas of dissatisfaction were highlighted. Financially, Donald felt his situation "couldn't be worse" and he drew a sharp contrast between his life before he was ill (when he was in full-time employment) and his current situation (living on benefits). Donald's health satisfaction was also quite low. He said the main problems were the voices, which were keeping him awake, and the side-effects of medication (even though he was no longer taking any). His self-esteem was very high - 10 positive responses out of 10.

Two Goal Attainment Scaling scales were worked out with Donald: to reduce the amount he heard voices and to start doing some voluntary work.

Six months later

In the six month period since the first interview, Donald had been in hospital. Initially detained under Section 2 (up to 28 days), he was then immediately detained under Section 3 (up to six months). Donald said that in retrospect he was "glad" that he had been put on a Section 2 but objected to the Section 3 which meant he could be taken back to hospital even though he was back in the community.

Donald was now taking two different medications and had put on even more weight (a total of seven stone), was still impotent and now suffered from leg tremors, agitation and photosensitivity. Donald was unhappy about taking medication and the effect it was having on him. He was still hearing voices. He said his community psychiatric nurse was trying to help him reduce one of the medications. He was still very unhappy about his relationship with his psychiatrist but was going to change to a different one soon (his third). Donald said he could not emphasise enough how short of beds and staff the hospital was:

> "I was very unhappy about the lack of beds - there is a severe shortage. In two weeks I was moved to six different wards. They had to put three beds in the Day Treatment Unit. In one week, five people slit their wrists or throats. Two were discharged in the same week and in days they were back in. Patients have been going as far as London."

Donald continued to try to attend the Hearing Voices group but often didn't have the money to get there (approximately 8 miles away).

Donald remained positive about his relationship with his community psychiatric nurse care manager. He had also been assigned a social worker and saw a member of the community mental health team every week. He commented:

> "I've always had a lot of faith in my CPN - I can't fault her."

Donald said that he still wanted his parent involved in his care, although to a lesser extent because he did not like her being responsible for him.

It seemed that because Donald's circumstances had changed quite significantly, his care programme was not just being reviewed, but completely revised. He said that the document had been printed but he did not want to sign it because he disagreed with some of it. He had agreed to keep seeing his community psychiatric nurse and social worker but commented:

> "... they want me to see a psychologist and have art therapy which I don't want."

He also said that he was refusing to sign the care programme until he had been given access to his medical records, which he has requested several times and which had not been forthcoming. When asked if the care programme addressed his needs he commented:

> "There should be more in the community. I would like to use decent facilities but there aren't any."

Although Donald was now doing the voluntary work he wanted, his work satisfaction on the Quality of Life measure had not increased: although he was pleased to be doing the voluntary work, he was unhappy that he was not being paid and was fearful that he would never be able to find full-time paid employment again because he is now labelled schizophrenic. Donald's leisure satisfaction had gone down due to his increasing frustration at having no money to spend on such activities and his financial satisfaction was still at the bottom of the scale. Donald's health score had not improved because he was still hearing voices (although to a lesser extent) and the effects of medication had worsened.

Summary

The CPA process had been partly successful for Donald. The relationship with his community psychiatric nurse was both strong and positive. He had been closely monitored and supported and his carer had been involved to the extent that he wished. On the negative side, Donald found community resources inadequate and he continued to have negative relationships with psychiatrists. He also felt pressurised to have services that he did not want and for this reason was refusing to sign the review document.

Carol: an unsuccessful care programme

Carol, a 40-year-old woman living with her husband and children, had been involved with services for over 20 years but had never been in hospital. She had been diagnosed as having depression. Carol said that she has been fighting for the past 20 years to get the support she needed.

Carol's care programme had been developed four months ago in response to her feeling more and more out of control of her life and things "getting too much". She was generally very positive about the care programme, but commented that it had only been in place a few months. When asked questions about feeling involved with services and professionals, Carol often commented that things were developing slowly and that it would take a long time for her to trust professionals. Carol said she felt she was being listened to and that everyone involved in the care programme was supportive (although she was disappointed when her psychiatrist left the care programme meeting after only a few minutes because he said he was busy).

Carol saw her community psychiatric nurse care manager once a week and the psychiatrist every month. Carol was very positive about her relationship with her care manager, feeling for the first time that they were "working together", but stated that she is always afraid that professionals will move on and she will be let down and have to build up relationships with new people. She also commented that she received a lot of support and help from community resources (ie, community centres, forum meetings, other support groups and social activities).

Carol stated that her husband was her main carer and that he was happy to be involved in the care programme, although she also emphasised that fact that he had a lot to cope with and that carers need support too. Carol was very keen for him to be part of the care programme and commented that he has not been formally involved in her mental health planning before.

From the problems/needs identified in the care programme, three Goal Attainment Scaling scales were worked out. Carol's aims were to reduce the extent to which she felt negative, depressed and anxious.

Carol's Quality of Life measure showed that she generally had mixed feelings about different aspects of her life. Her self-esteem was very low - 10 negative responses out of a possible 10. It was agreed that the self-esteem score would provide a good way of measuring the impact of the self-esteem building group she was to attend as part of her care programme.

Six months later

At Survey One Carol felt she had some say in planning her mental healthcare but at Survey Two she that that she definitely did not. She said that the care programme had been reviewed about a month ago and at this meeting her and her husband were told that her care manager would be away for a year doing a course. They were told that there would be no one available to take his place. Apparently, her care manager had requested that Carol have regular support from a social worker but had been told that, due to lack of resources, staff were only being assigned to users coming out of hospital. Carol commented:

> "Staff at the mental health centre have gone and the psychiatrist is leaving. No one knows if these people will be replaced ... it makes a mockery out of the care programme."

Carol said that she had a care programme in theory but not in practice. She commented that her husband was also affected by this:

> "It's very hard for him to cope sometimes - he's not got any back up."

Carol felt that because her husband cared for her and she was not "in crisis" (ie, likely to be admitted to hospital very soon), she was being ignored. However, Carol stated that she really felt she needed support and regular contact at the moment: she had recently found out that she had a serious medical condition. Carol commented:

> "I get most of my support from my friends here [community centre run by MIND] but they've got mental health problems too. I talk but I don't want to burden them, it's not fair on them - they've got their own problems."

Carol said she had been positive and optimistic about the care and support she had received through the care programme until she found out that she would not have a care manager for a year. She still attended support groups run by voluntary services and one run at the mental health centre. She had to conclude that the care programme had not worked out well because:

> "It's good in theory but not in practice. The care programme made me feel there was someone there - now there's no one-to-one."

Carol said that she had a number to call at the hospital if she needed someone to talk to but said that talking to a stranger could never replace communicating with someone she trusted and had built up a relationship with. Carol was still very positive about her care manager, feeling very comfortable with him and finding him very respectful to her.

There had been some changes in Carol's Quality of Life measure scores since Survey One. Carol felt more satisfied with not being in employment at the second interview and commented that she was relieved that she was not working because she felt that she would not be able to cope in her current circumstances (particularly the extra worry caused by her illness). Carol was less satisfied with her leisure activities, commenting that her illness, the withdrawal of her care manager and a problem one of her children was having at school had made her:

> "... so worried about everything I can't enjoy myself."

Carol's health score was down one point reflecting that she was less satisfied with both her physical and mental health.

Looking at the Goal Attainment Scaling, Carol said her negative thoughts were the same, but that her depression and anxiety had reduced slightly (she attributed this to her own efforts). Carol's self-esteem was still extremely low. She said that the member of the community mental health team who had run the self-esteem group for a few weeks had had a breakdown due to workload pressures and had ended up in psychiatric hospital. She also commented that staff who were leaving were not being replaced.

Summary

Carol's worst fears, expressed in the first interview, had been realised by the time of the second interview six months later. She was tentatively positive about the care programme in Survey One but expressed a fear that her care manager would change and she would have to build up a relationship with someone new. By Survey Two she had no care manager at all (at least for a year). During Survey One she commented that the best thing about the care programme was that it was a recognition that she needed help. By Survey Two she felt she was being left to cope on her own. Both Carol and her husband felt very disappointed and frustrated. Carol said she really needed support during this difficult time in her life - she was scared of her physical illness and its psychological consequences. She felt that she would only get help if she "did something silly" and ended up in hospital. Support from her husband and the need to try and carry on for the sake of her children made Carol cope, but sometimes she just felt like "giving up" or "ending it all". She concluded:

> "There needs to be a lot of changes - the government gives you something with one hand and then takes it away with the other."

Robert: a user without a care programme

Robert, in early middle-age and living with his wife and children, had been in hospital three times in the last five years, suffering from depression, but had never been sectioned. He stated that he had definitely not been asked if he wanted his carer, his wife, involved in planning his care, even though he definitely wanted her involved. He felt unable to say what his problems and needs were to professionals and had not been asked what he thought about his admissions to hospital or involvement with services. He did not have a care manager. Robert said that he had not been given information on any of the eight rights and services listed. Overall, he concluded that he was not satisfied with the service he was receiving.

Robert's wife, Christine, said she wanted to be involved in her husband's care to some extent but had not really been asked. She was unsure as to whether or not she had been encouraged to say what her aims were for Robert's care and treatment and felt she had been asked her opinions on his hospital admissions and involvement with services a little. She also stated that he did not have a care manager and that she had not been given information on any of the rights and services listed. Overall, she felt she felt she had little say in her husband's mental healthcare planning and she was only marginally satisfied with services.

Six months later

Robert's responses to the questions were very similar to the ones he gave in the first interview. He commented that he still did not have a care manager but that he would like to see someone regularly. He felt he had nowhere to go and nothing to do and would enjoy having a purposeful day activity. Again, he said that he had not been asked if he wanted his wife involved in his care because:

> "It is just assumed that she will take care of me."

Robert stated that he definitely wanted her involved in his care and that she always went with him to the see the GP or psychiatrist - the only two health professionals they had regular contact with. When asked if he felt encouraged by professionals to say what his problems and needs were, Robert commented:

> "I don't see any professionals from the mental health team. I only see the psychiatrist or GP about medication."

Many of the questions in the interview seemed irrelevant to Robert because he actually had no contact with the community mental health team, despite being eligible for a care programme. When asked what he liked most and least about the service being received, Robert commented:

"I don't really think I'm receiving a service."

Robert said that he was not satisfied with services and wished he had the option of having regular contact with a member of the community mental health team and had information on the sort of services and support available.

Christine commented that she had never been asked about her own needs and had not been asked if she wanted to be involved in Robert's care:

> "They just assume that because I cope well they don't need to see us. They don't even ask me what I think. I've been told many times by professionals that my problem is that I 'cope too well'."

When asked if she wanted to be involved in her husband's care, Christine commented:

> "I absolutely want to help Robert but regular support from a professional would help - perhaps me more than it would him."

Christine said she was very happy with their relationships with the GP and psychiatrist but commented that there was no real support for Robert, herself or their children. She commented on not being aware of what services, support or community resources were available for either of them.

Summary

Although happy with the service being provided by the GP and psychiatrist, both Robert and his carer Christine wanted regular support from the community mental health team. Neither had heard of care programmes and Robert did not have a care manager. Their responses during the first and second interviews were very similar and generally negative. Both felt isolated, unsupported and were unaware of what services, both statutory and voluntary, were available to them.

11

Discussion and conclusions

The project has demonstrated that mental health services can be more responsive to the needs of people with severe and long-term mental health problems. An approach to care management, care programming, was developed with the goal of involving users and carers in assessing needs and planning care and treatment in the community. The approach was developed in collaboration with users and carers in an area which was close to the national average in terms of the incidence of social problems associated with mental ill-health. The mental health service was under significant pressure from lack of resources and no special funding was available for increased service provision. These are grounds to believe that, given the commitment of managers and staff, the same effects could be replicated elsewhere.

The results of the evaluation showed that users with care programmes felt more involved in planning their own care and treatment, had more choice and were better informed about rights and services compared to similar group of users without care programmes. Over three quarters of users agreed with their care programmes, thought that they were clear and comprehensive and that the care programme addressed their needs.

Users and carers were positive about their relationships with community-based care managers, community psychiatric nurses or social workers. In their opinion, a stable, trusting relationship with one professional enhanced service delivery and continuity of care. This finding is consistent with results from a number of studies of care management in mental health services (Onyett, 1992).

The picture which emerged was that users felt positive and comfortable with more 'holistic', community-based services, rather than 'medical', hospital-based ones. Users felt they had much more choice in their care and treatment in the community rather than hospital and they were more likely to agree with their care manager about their problems and needs than their psychiatrist. Of course, in the case of users 'on Section' of the Mental Health Act, there is little or no choice available and the potential for user involvement is decidedly limited. The majority of the personal goals worked out by users for Goal Attainment Scaling were of practical or social nature, rather than psychological/psychiatric. These findings imply that the CPA is more in line with what users want from services compared to solely medical-based models of mental healthcare provision. It is important to remember that the users surveyed were experienced recipients of inpatient and community services with enduring and/or severe mental health problems. They experienced a greater degree of social isolation than the rest of the population with nearly half living alone and one in five living in residential care. Over a quarter said they had no carer and over one third specified a professional as their main carer. The more complex levels of the CPA were designed to provide monitoring and support in the community for the sort of users who took part in the project and findings demonstrated that the main aims and principles of this approach were practicable and successful for these users.

The approach to user involvement employed in the project was grounded in a formal procedure, care programming. Formal procedures can sometimes create barriers to forming the relationships which are an essential part of enabling involvement (Ellis, 1993; Stevenson and Parsloe, 1993). However, in mental health services it may be that formal procedures which emphasise users' views (for example the requirement to record users' views on the care programme forms) are a necessary element in countering the prevailing power relationships in favour of mental health professionals. It is important to remember that the group of users who did not have care programmes were nevertheless on the caseloads of the community mental health teams and/or the consultant psychiatrists. The differences we found between the groups can therefore be attributed to the effects of having a care programme and, we argue, the elements within that process which were designed to promote involvement and empowerment. The evidence of these differences effectively contradicts the belief of at least some professionals that "We're doing it all already" (Marsh and Fisher, 1992).

Among the obstacles to effective involvement is lack of information (Baldock and Ungerson, 1994). Without information about rights and services, users are in a poor position to make choices. We found that, even though the care programme procedures did effect an improvement in users' knowledge, there were still significant gaps. This was noticeably evident in relation to information about alternatives to medication and knowledge about complaints procedures (Sbaraini and Carpenter, 1996a). Regardless of whether they had care programmes, many users were poorly informed about rights and services, had thought about making a complaint about services, and felt they had little choice in their care and treatment in hospital, and so on. Users expressed the power imbalances they felt in their relationships with services. The issue of complaints highlighted this, with many users expressing fears that, if they did complain, services might be withdrawn or imposed.

Previous research on community care has suggested that users and carers needs might often conflict (Ellis, 1993; Stevenson and Parsloe, 1993). We found that, on the whole, users and their carers tended to agree rather than disagree with each other about the users' needs. Initially, three quarters of users wanted their carers involved in planning their care but six months later, they were less likely to report that their carers were involved; they were also less likely to want them involved. Further, the carers we interviewed wanted to be involved in their relatives' care. We found that carers tended to feel less involved after the initial care programme meetings. Carers' own needs were rarely considered by professionals. It seems that with the focus very firmly on the, often considerable, needs of the user, conflicts were probably under emphasised in care programming.

Does involvement lead to empowerment? Any experience of empowerment in the care programming process might be more in the eye of the beholder and in any case turn out to be short lived. Certainly most of the users who responded to our questions felt involved and empowered to take part in the care programming process. Further, two thirds considered that their care programme had worked out well, or very well. However, as the case profiles illustrate, empowerment is fragile. In most cases, 10 out of the 17 which we followed up, the positive experiences had been retained, but in others, the outcome had been mixed, and in a few the breakdown in care had led to disillusionment. Both users and carers recognised the effect of resource constraints on care and treatment and levels of support. A good mental health service enables users to be less dependent on it when their mental health improves. However, many users and carers expressed fears about support being removed prematurely and a number felt this had already happened.

Finally, we should note the impact of the project and its evaluation on the local mental health service. The profile of the CPA had been raised and its potential for user and carer involvement at least partly realised. In the opinion of the professionals, there had been benefits for multidisciplinary team working and the service managers reported considerably improved working relationships between the hospital and community-based staff. The managers acted on the findings as they emerged, developing interagency information systems, devising an information pack for users, setting up an audit and successfully arguing for increased staff resources for care programming from the health authority. The number of care programmes developed with and for people with severe and long-term problems has more than tripled in the last few months. The project has been fully absorbed by the mental health system and we can feel optimistic that the improvements will endure so long as the principles in which the approach was grounded remain in people's minds. This will require continuing review and the induction of new staff, users and carers, into the values as well as the procedures, for the mechanisms of participation cannot guarantee that it will actually take place.

References and further reading

Audit Commission (1994) *Finding a place: a review of mental health services for adults,* London: HMSO.

Baldock, J. and Ungerson, C. (1994) *Becoming consumers of community care: households within a mixed economy of welfare,* York: Joseph Rowntree Foundation.

Berforth, M., Conlan, E., Field, V., Hoser, B. and Syce, L. (eds) (1990) *Whose service is it anyway? Users' views on co-ordinating community care,* London: Research and Development in Psychiatry.

Burns, T., Beardsmore, A., Bhat, A.V., Oliver, A. and Mathers, C. (1993) 'A controlled trial of home-based acute psychiatric services', *British Journal of Psychiatry,* vol 163, pp 49-54.

Campbell, P. (1992) 'A survivor's view of community psychiatry', *Journal of Mental Health,* vol 1, pp 117-22.

Carpenter, J. and Sbaraini, S. (1996) 'Involving users and carers in the Care Programme Approach', *Journal of Mental Health,* vol 5, no 5, pp 483-88.

Department of Health (1990) *The Care Programme Approach,* HC(90)23/LASSL(90)11, London: DoH.

Department of Health (1994) *The Health of the Nation key area handbook: mental illness,* Heywood: BAPS Health Publications Unit.

Department of Health (1995) *Building bridges: a guide to arrangements for inter-agency working for the care and protection of severely mentally ill people,* London: DoH.

District Audit (1995) *Mental health audit 1994/95, Canterbury and Thanet Community Healthcare Trust.*

Ellis, K. (1993) *Squaring the circle. User and carer participation in needs assessment,* York: Joseph Rowntree Foundation.

Hansson, L. (1989) 'Patient satisfaction with in-hospital psychiatric care', *European Archives of Psychiatry and Neurological Sciences,* vol 239, pp 93-100.

Holly, L. and Webb, B. (1993) *Citizen advocacy in practice: the experience of the Scarborough-Ryedale-Whitby Advocacy Alliance,* London: The Tavistock Institute.

Kiresek, T., Smith, A. and Cardillo, J. (eds) (1994) *Goal attainment scaling: applications, theory and measurement,* Hillsdale, NJ: Lawrence Earlbaum.

Lindow, V. and Morris, J. (1995) *Service user involvement. Synthesis of findings and experience in the field of community care,* York: Joseph Rowntree Foundation.

Marsh, P. and Fisher, M. (1992) *Good intentions: developing partnership in social services,* York: Joseph Rowntree Foundation.

Merson, S., Tyrer, P., Onyett, S.R., Lynch, S., Lack, S. and Johnson, A.L. (1992) 'Early intervention in psychiatric emergencies: a controlled clinical trial', *Lancet,* vol 339, pp 1311-14.

Muijen, M., Marks, I., Connolly, J. and Audini, B. (1992) 'Home based and standard hospital care for patients with severe mental illness: a randomised controlled trial', *British Medical Journal,* vol 304, pp 749-54.

North, C., Ritchie, J. and Ward, K. (1993) *Factors influencing the implementation of the Care Programme Approach,* London: HMSO.

Oliver, J. et al (1995) *Quality of Life and mental health services,* London: Routledge.

Onyett, S.R. (1992) *Case management in mental health,* London: Chapman & Hall.

Onyett, S.R., Pillinger, T. and Muijen, M. (1995) *Making community mental health teams work,* London: Sainsbury Centre for Mental Health.

Rogers, A. and Pilgrim, D. (1991) 'Pulling down churches: accounting for the British mental health users' movement', *Sociology of Health and Illness,* vol 13, pp 129-48.

Sbaraini, S. and Carpenter, J. (1996a) 'Barriers to complaints: a survey of mental health users', *Journal of Management in Medicine,* vol 10, no 6, pp 37-41.

Sbaraini, S. and Carpenter, J. (1996b) *GPs and the Care Programme Approach: report of a survey,* Canterbury: Tizard Centre, University of Kent.

Schneider, J., Hayes, L., Beecham, J. and Knapp, M. (1993) *Care programming in mental health: a study of implementation and costs in three health districts,* PSSRU Discussion Paper 922/2, Canterbury: University of Kent.

Social Services Inspectorate/Department of Health (1995) *Social services department and the Care Programme Approach,* London: SSI/DoH, p 4.

Stevenson, O. and Parsloe, P. (1993) *Community care and empowerment,* York: Joseph Rowntree Foundation.

[In addition to this report, the authors have written and distributed a number of reports in the local area. They have also written two papers in academic journals and others are in preparation.]

Appendix A - Research tools and methods

User questionnaire

The user questionnaire/structured interview schedule was developed in consultation with local user and carer representatives using a focus group method. The questionnaire contained a number of sections designed to investigate involvement, empowerment and the extent to which users felt the various 'quality standards' outlined by the trust had been met in their own care and treatment.

Each section of the questionnaire typically included a number of set questions, with a 5-point forced answer type scale, and spaces for comments. Relevant 'background information' was also collected in the questionnaires, that is, age, sex, time involved with services, number of hospital admissions, and so on. The user questionnaire was used as a self-complete postal questionnaire and interview schedule for Surveys One and Two.

Details of the statistical tests used to compare differences between groups may be found in Carpenter and Sbaraini (1996).

Carer questionnaire

The carer questionnaire/structured interview schedule contained equivalent questions to those in the user questionnaire. For example, where users were asked, "Do you want your carer involved in your care planning?", carers were asked, "Do you want to be involved in your relative's care planning?" The carer questionnaire was used as a self-complete postal questionnaire and interview schedule for Surveys One and Two.

Peer interviewing materials

User and carer peer interviewers used the user and carer questionnaires. A number of other materials/documents were also developed:

The 'notes for interviewers' were given to peer interviewers during the training sessions. These included a brief description of the research, general guidelines (on, for example, interview techniques, confidentiality, safety) and procedures for arranging the interviews.

A 'letter of identification' was provided for each interviewer and was designed to be shown to the interviewee before the interview. The letter included a brief description of the project and how interviewees were invited to take part, the name of the interviewer and the dates between which they would be doing interviews, and a contact name, address and number. The letters were signed and dated by the project director.

A 'post-interview sheet' was given to all interviewees, after they had been interviewed, by the interviewer. This included the name of the interviewer, a brief description of the project and a contact name, address and telephone number in case of any questions of queries.

A 'post-interview comments and check sheet' was completed by the interviewers after each interview. It included a space for the interviewers to include any comments and a number of questions designed to check that the interviewing procedures had been followed, that is, that the interviewee had been paid and had been given a post-interview sheet.

Goal Attainment Scaling

This outcome measure, devised by Kiresek and Sherman in the United States (Kiresek, Smith and Cardillo, 1994) is based on the development and scaling of personal goals. Problems or needs identified by the user in their care programme were discussed with the researcher and a way of measuring improvement or deterioration in that area was worked out. See below for an example of how the personal goal of 'doing some voluntary work' was measured.

Level of attainment:	Attainment level +3	Attainment level +2	Attainment level +1	Current status 0	Attainment level -1
Scale 1: to do some voluntary work	Does three or more sessions/days per week	Does two sessions/days per week	Does one session/day per week	Does no voluntary work	No longer wants to do voluntary work

Goal Attainment Scaling scales were worked out with users at Survey One and the level of attainment assessed six months later at Survey Two. At Survey One the user would always be at the 'current status 0' level. At Survey Two the user could be at any attainment level from -1 to +3, including 0.

Goal Attainment Scaling was used to provide a way of measuring the effect of care programmes on outcomes for users.

Lancashire Quality of Life measure

This structured interview schedule was designed by Oliver et al (1995) to assess the user's quality of life. It examines a number of different life areas: work/education, leisure, religion, finances, living situation, legal and safety, family relations, social relations and health. It also includes a general life satisfaction scale and a self-esteem measure. Users assess each life area by replying to a number of questions on a fixed 7-point scale:

1	2	3	4	5	6	7
Couldn't be worse	Very unsatisfied	Quite unsatisfied	Mixed (about equally satisfied and unsatisfied)	Quite satisfied	Very satisfied	Couldn't be better

Self-esteem is measured by users either agreeing or disagreeing with 5 positive and 5 negative statements about themselves. 0 represents the lowest self-esteem (ie, the user agreed with all 5 negative statements and disagreed with all 5 positive ones) and 10 represents the highest self-esteem (ie, the user disagreed with all 5 negative statements and agreed with all 5 positive).

The Quality of Life schedule was given to users with care programmes by the researcher at Survey One and then six months later at Survey Two. It was used to assess the impact of care programmes on different areas of users' life satisfaction.

Professional questionnaire

The professional questionnaire used in the staff survey was a self-complete questionnaire containing open ended questions, set questions with 5-point forced type answer scales, comments sections and a number of statements with which professionals either agreed or disagreed.

The questionnaire was designed to identify what professionals perceived to be the costs and rewards of the CPA and examined whether or not they thought it would have a positive or negative effect on some key areas including, user and carer involvement, multidisciplinary teamwork, and administration.

The first staff survey was completed just after CPA training and the follow-up survey was completed approximately six months later. The surveys provided a measure of staff attitudes and experiences over time.

GP questionnaire

The GP questionnaire was developed to include relevant questions that had been used in other GP surveys (ie, "Who should be responsible for the monitoring of patients?") as well as others designed to investigate attitudes user and carer involvement and the tiered CPA. The questionnaire also contained background information questions, such as GPs' contact with mental health workers, experience in psychiatric posts, use of counsellors in surgeries. Fixed response questions were used to assess knowledge of and attitudes to the CPA and the care and treatment of patients with mental health problems. The GP questionnaire was used in a single postal survey. (See Sbaraini and Carpenter, 1996b.)

Appendix B: Care Programme Approach form

Canterbury and Thanet Community Health Care Trust
and
Kent Social Services Department
Care programme

Date of meeting(s):

Name:
Address:

Post code:
Tel no:
Date of birth:
Living with:

Main carer
Name:
Address:

Post code:
Tel no:

Care manager
Name:
Address:

Post code:
Tel no:

Reason for programme
Sec. 117 ☐
3+ hospital admissions ☐
Other ☐

Date of admission:
Sec. of Mental Health Act
2, 3, 37, 41, 47, 48 (*circle*)

GP
Name:
Address:

Post code:
Tel no:

Consultant
Name:

Other people and agencies involved

Name	Agency/ relationship	Address	Tel no

Copies of this programme to be sent to: *(please tick)*

Client	Carer	GP	Hospital notes	Outpatients	Team manager	Other

Referral and involvement

(1) Client's views

On referral or admission to hospital:

On having a care programme:

On involvement of carers and family:

Would client like an advocate?

(2) **Carers' views**
     On involvement with client's problems/needs:

     Support they are able to provide:

     Does carer want an assessment of own needs?

(3) **Care manager's comments** (including action to be taken on above information)

Needs/problems identified

Areas for consideration	Problem/need identified by			
	Client	Carer	Case manager	Key worker
Getting on with others *(family, partner, friends, at work)*				
Psychological/psychiatric symptoms *(eg, depression, anxiety, hallucinations)*				
Looking after yourself *(including appearance, physical health)*				
Accommodation *(including personal safety)*				
Money *(including benefits)*				
Social support, spiritual needs and recreation				
Employment and day activities *(including voluntary work, education)*				
Anything else *(eg, legal problems, alcohol and drug problem)*				

Care plan

*Please complete a **separate** sheet for each type of problem or need noted above.*

Medication	
Current medication:	Injection treatment arrangement: CPN Clinic GP Repeat prescription arrangements: GP Outpatients
Have possible side-effects been explained? When will medication be reviewed? How? *(please circle)* GP Outpatients Home visit Doctor's initials	

Arrangement for monitoring and reviewing this plan

Monitoring *(to check that the plan is being put into action)*
Date of next meeting between client and care manager:

Review
Date of meeting: Where:

Who should be invited:

Information given

Rights with respect to Mental Health Act *(where appropriate)* ☐	Local user forum ☐
Right not to have a care programme ☐	Effects of medication, including side-effects ☐
	Pharmacy helpline ☐
What to do if dissatisfied *(contact the team manager in the first instance)* ☐	Duty system (Community mental health team) ☐
Formal complaints procedure ☐	Out of hours services ☐
Access to records ☐	How to contact other services ☐
Advocacy service ☐	Welfare rights advice ☐

Agreement

I have discussed this care plan and my views are given above. I agree with the actions proposed.

Signatures

Client .... Carer (if appropriate) ....

Care manager ....

Date ....

Example (names and details have been changed)

Care plan

Please state which problem/type of need:
Personal hygiene/physical health

Views of	Problem/need	Aims	Action	Who by	Unmet
Client Zoe	I sometimes need help in washing and dressing myself. I sometimes need help to choose my clothes each day.	To look pretty and feel good.	1. Key worker/staff member helps me to wash shower etc. 2. Key worker/staff member helps me to choose my clothes each day. 3. I tell Joyce when I feel poorly	Zoe Zoe Zoe	
Carer Joyce	Zoe needs help with personal hygiene. Zoe requires support when physically unwell. Zoe needs help in choosing clothing appropriate to the season eg Zoe may wear thick jumpers on a hot day.	1. For Zoe to look and feel presentable and comfortable. 2. For Zoe to remain physically well. 3. For Zoe to become more independent in personal hygiene, physical health and choosing her own clothes	1. Remind Zoe to wash/bathe/shower daily with support. 2. Remind Zoe to change clothes/ underwear daily. 3. Help with washing hair and care of hair, nails and teeth. 4. Arrange appointments with GP. 5. Help Zoe to choose clothing appropriate to the season.	Joyce Joyce Joyce/ chiropody/ hairdresser Joyce Joyce	
Care manager Laura (CPN)	Monitor physical health for any deterioration	As above	1. Offer health education to Zoe and carers. 2. Observe and report any signs of physical illness to carers and involve GP. 3. Monitor personal hygiene, etc and offer advice and support to Zoe and carers.	Laura Laura Laura	

Appendix C: Care Programme Approach training workshop: a case study

John Fredericks (24 years old) is well known to the local mental health services, having had two short-term hospital admissions during the last 18 months. On each occasion, John had been a voluntary patient and discharged himself back to his family home.

Two weeks ago he was picked up by the police for creating a nuisance - he was standing in the middle of the road directing traffic. Since he refused to move on and he appeared to be having delusions, the police requested a psychiatric assessment. John refused to speak at any length to either the psychiatrist or the approved social worker and declined to go into hospital. The psychiatrist recommended his admission under Section 2 of the Mental Health Act on the grounds that he was suffering from a mental illness and that he should be detained in the interests of his own safety. He has been diagnosed as having schizophrenia.

John, an only child, was living with his mother and stepfather, Mrs and Mr Tanner. His mother had previously told the community psychiatric nurse who had been visiting the family at home that she felt very sorry for her son whose father had left when he was two years old. She had tried to "make it up to him" by giving him the very best that she could afford and always tried to understand his difficult behaviour.

Things had gradually become even more difficult over the last three years. John and his stepfather did not get on well together. Mr Tanner had married his wife eight years before (when John was 16), and had always left dealings with John up to his wife. However, he had become increasingly angry at John's treatment of his mother, and complained that she let John treat her like a servant, abusing her verbally, demanding food at all hours and expecting her to pay for his frequent nights out. He was incensed that John lost his job in a warehouse because "he couldn't be bothered with the bus journey".

On a visit to the hospital, Mrs Tanner told John's key worker on the ward that her husband would be even more angry if he found out that she had been selling her jewellery to pay for John's drinking *and* drawn a substantial sum (£350) from their joint savings account to settle some of his debts).

Since his admission, John had been taking medication under duress. He didn't consider that he had a mental illness and at the ward meeting he told the psychiatrist that he was quite happy living at home and wanted to return there. He didn't think that there were any problems there. His only need was for a good job, that is, one which paid him a decent wage, but in the meantime his mother would go on lending him what he needed.

John meets the criteria for the CPA. How would you advise the key worker or the care manager to go about setting up a meeting? Remember that the task is not to sort out all his problems in one go, but rather to develop a care programme for his aftercare.